T0354411

NO TIME FOR DIETS

L. Raynes MS.RDN.CDE.

authorHOUSE®

AuthorHouse™ LLC
1663 Liberty Drive
Bloomington, IN 47403
www.authorhouse.com
Phone: 1-800-839-8640

Published by AuthorHouse 08/29/2014

ISBN: 978-1-4969-3111-5 (sc)
ISBN: 978-1-4969-3079-8 (hc)
ISBN: 978-1-4969-3113-9 (e)

Library of Congress Control Number: 2014913750

Did you know that obesity is the greatest single preventable cause of death in the United States? Yet according to the CDC in 2014, 78.6 million adults are obese. Two thirds of Americans are either overweight or obese. One third of Americans are obese today compared to 23% in the 1980s. The average American male is 18% overweight, and the average American female is 27% overweight. Further obesity is becoming the new norm. The world has recently been introduced to the "fatkini". The odds of you becoming obese rise to 57% if your friend is obese, and 40% if you have a sibling who is obese according to the New England Journal of Medicine in 2009. The internet, television, movies, and ads proclaim that thin is in. But nutrition education has never been one of the three R's. So, health conscious, overweight Americans listen to any and all advice on how to make molehills out of their mountains, no matter whether the information is inaccurate, incomplete or totally erroneous. In fact, over 30,000 methods of weight control contribute to the multi-billion dollar diet industry. Sadly, however, over half of these methods are backed by nutrition fraud, misinformation, and fad diets. It's time for a book on weight control that works!

It's time for you to do something for the health of it! Here, at last is guidance flexible enough to work into any lifestyle, whether you have tried unsuccessfully to lose weight, again and again. If you have other health issues or your life is stress filled, have heart diseases or diabetes, no matter how hectic your lifestyle is, this will enable you to live a healthier life, and become the weight you want to be for now as well as tomorrow. Yes, "No Time for Diets" is not only a workable program but one that is nutritionally balanced and an economical alternative, adaptable to even the most sophisticated palate. To tell the world that there is no miracle solution or short cut is to destroy the American dream. To offer a workable solution that can be tailored to any individuals' automated "no time" lifestyle can spell creative success.

Simple nutrition principles, accurately applied spell the difference between uncontrolled weight gain, and finally obesity, or healthy, effective weight control.

GENERAL COVERAGE:

"No Time for Diets" is less about diets and more about understanding what goals you want to set and how to achieve them to achieve permanent weight loss and control. It helps you understand your calorie budget. Then it shows you how to budget your calorie salary by offering practical, working knowledge of nutrition principles. This is vital for total weight management. It combines these principles with guidelines that are flexible enough to fit into any individual lifestyle for successful weight control.

CREDENTIALS:

I am a registered dietitian/nutritionist with a master's of science degree in Food and Nutrition. I am also board certified as a diabetes educator. Currently, I am an active member of the Academy of Nutrition and Dietetics and have been registered since 1973. I have also been a member to the following specialty groups; Weight Management, Renal Specialty, Diabetes Care and Education Practice Group, Consultant Nutritionists in Private Practice, and have been a member of the National Kidney Foundation, American Diabetes Association, ASPEN, and the American Heart Association. In each of the settings I have worked closely with weight reduction in groups, and individuals with good success. I have developed and taught nutrition classes for the University of Maryland, Lawrence Memorial School of Nursing, in Massachusetts, Sarasota Memorial Hospital Weight Management Center, Manatee Junior College, and the Longboat Key Adult Education Center in Florida. Over the years, I have spoken at various forums and seminars on nutrition and weight management. I have appeared on television programs to discuss weight management and nutrition, have been interviewed, and written for newspapers, as well as contributing to a weekly newspaper column. I am a published author in both nonscientific publications as well as peer reviewed publication of the renal dietetics practice group. The most recent article was co-authored and published in the Renal Nutrition Forum Volume 32, Number 2, entitled "Nutritional Consequences and Benefits of Alternatives to In-Center Hemodialysis".

Finally, what makes this most credible is the fact that I am currently the owner of a successful website, www.notimefordiets.com. This website provides ongoing support to people interested in a healthy lifestyle. It helps you apply principles in this "no time for a balanced diet" world and do it for the health of it. Even in a high stress position, with virtually, no defined working hours, these principles work! I want to invite you too to do it for the health of it!

TABLE OF CONTENTS

First things first, motivation is a key ingredient in your quest for successful weight reduction. This chapter tests not only the reader's desire, but the environment to get set for success. A mind set for success, cannot fail, when trained to stay on track. Motivational cueing is discussed, to be certain that you want to do exactly what it is you have set out to do. There are undeniable outside influences, and the timing must be right for success. Knowing thyself and your lifestyle can lead to the wonderful realization that today is the time to take control of your lifestyle.

To be successful, you must set a specific goal, and perhaps more importantly, see yourself reaching that specific weight goal. Visualization is a powerful tool that can be put to work. To set a goal you must have a specific aim in mind. Secondly, you must know exactly when you will reach your plateaus. Finally you must outline the steps that you will take to reach that goal. Steps to reach that final goal with the intermediate goals along the way are developed.

As the breadbasket of the world, we have too much food to choose from. Couple this with insufficient knowledge to make the most healthful choices, and the combination can add up to tons of excess fat and effective dietary suicide. Most weight reducers enormously underestimate the number of calories that they eat in a day. More, we tend to overestimate the number of calories that we burn up. Calorie concepts are explained in detail to set the groundwork for keeping in touch with the foods that make up the person. Food diaries with their pros and cons are introduced and detailed explanations of this tool and the use of group foods are discussed.

This chapter concentrates on what you can do to avoid daily obstacles with preplans. "No Time for Diets" focuses on personal motivation, coupled with the appropriate preplanned choices, to enable you to set self selected goals while avoiding the stumbling blocks that discourage and frustrate. Focusing on what you can do, personally, today is the key.

You don't have to join a health club, jog two miles a day, or swim laps in a pool to get the activity to help your new body look its best. What you do need to do is have a general idea of what is going to happen to you and what it will do to your planning. Exercise, as an adjunct to the loss of fat mass, is discussed, and a plan to increase exercise that is fun is outlined and encouraged.

Armed with only good intentions isn't' enough. The take-charge arrangements must take place where you spend the most time. The work place is full of sabotage situations, and excuses for "just this once". Successful people are able to keep a positive mental attitude to break down the barriers that are keeping you from your thin self. The role of a supporting cast is introduced and discussed with emphasis on the responsibility for weight management in today's world. Food facts and alternate plans of attack will keep you on the road to success whether you want to lose that evasive ten pounds or one hundred.

The sheer will power to say, "no" is never enough. Here are some practical suggestions when you have failed to plan or circumstances have not worked in your favor and as a result you are "starving". These techniques are provided to give you ammunition when you have no time and all the good intentions. Safe snacks are also included.

It's easy to be overwhelmed by the barrage of advertisements that claim miracle weight loss. Our automated society gets work done rapidly and without pain. We want the same magic in our own weight management. The American quest for slimness has led to over 30,000 methods of weight control, proliferated, in part, by the failure of most manufacturers to provide timely information. This is a practical guide to label reading that tells what to look for on a nutrition label, and what it tells you when the information is NOT there.

Think... before opening the refrigerator and your mouth trap. This chapter will help you learn to control your eating responses. The very "learned" responses to advertisements that sponsor count on, and the sight of food, can be unlearned too. This is how the media manages to promote junk foods. Learn to spot the cues. Then changing your channel will make YOU, not the advertiser, the winner.

To continue to be successful, you must make it as easy as possible. What is easy for us, we will continue to do. Whatever is difficult, we will change. This chapter focuses on giving you power in your world. Placement of foods in the kitchen and safe snacks are important aspects of increasing your "willpower". Sodium and its problems are elaborated upon, as well as the use of supplements, particularly calcium, fish oils, and cholesterol, binge foods, and health foods.

CHAPTER 11: CANDLELIGHT FOR TWO...VICTORY
Deprivation is your enemy. Just because you are losing weight, is no reason not to celebrate. Holidays and restaurant dining offer special challenges. Information and format activities for handling these special occasions make this a WIN-WIN situation. Alcohol, as a stumbling block is discussed as well as its use.

Linda A. Raynes Mahony, M.S.RDN. CDE.
www.notimefordiets.com

Chapter 1

Check Your Mind Set
Blueprint for Success

This is a game of mind over matter. What you think matters. In fact, motivation is the single most important ingredient in your successful weight management program. If you are interested in weight loss and permanent control it is you who must take the first and most important step in exerting control in your environment. This chapter will check your desire as well as the environmental role in your ultimate success.

Obesity has become the greatest single preventable cause of death in the United States. Well known consequences of obesity include hypertension, dyslipidemia, diabetes, cardiovascular disease, stroke, sleep apnea, osteoarthritis, respiratory problems, liver disease, as well as increased risk of endometrial, breast, prostrate and colon cancers. The total costs attributable to all obesity related diseases have continued to rise, and have approached $190.2 billion in the United States in the past years or 21% of our annual medical spending. In fact, childhood obesity costs alone are $14 billion dollars. Yet, according to the National Health and Nutrition Examination Survey more than two thirds of Americans either remain overweight or obese. According to the experts, obesity is not only an epidemic, in this country it is a global explosion! The cause of the obesity epidemic is not only because of our automated society, although that is part of it. We certainly use fewer Calories in physical activity then we did when we were a more agrarian society. We no longer milk cows by hand, nor plant fields and harvest them manually. We don't chop woods or split it. We don't have to build a fire to keep us warm or walk to town to pick up supplies. We don't wash our clothes manually, nor do we even iron the clothes after laundering for the most part. We don't have to know how to cook our food because everything is pre packaged, frozen, processed. All we really know how to do is press the quick start on the microwave, or go to a fast food restaurant or other eatery to be fed. The carrots are pre peeled. The vegetables can be purchased, all canned or frozen. We don't have to carry water to the house, nor do we need to worry about even walking down to the mailbox for the most part, because of the internet and online everything! We watch television, or spend time on the computer, check our voice or email, and watch sports instead of participating in them. Our children don't have to walk to school. There are buses for that, or their parents drive them. We are surrounded by mechanical and electronic inventions to assure that we do as little physical activity as possible. We don't get up to change the channel of the television. We use a remote control. We seldom even wash the dishes. There are, after all dishwashers for that. We have even added powered golf carts to golf so we don't have to "walk the course". In fact, there are some golf courses that insist you rent a cart if you want to play golf or require that you pay for and use a caddy. And despite all of these automations, when I ask people what kind of activities they do, probably nine times out of ten the people will say, "I'm active all day!" But with a little more investigation less then 10% of the people will walk 10,000 steps in a day!

Today, in the bread basket of the world, we are under the intense marketing pressure from manufacturers, in a fiercely competitive war all vying for our dollars. We are inundated with slogans to purchase fast food that we can have, "our way". But then, we have to decide if "the burgers are better". Manufacturers are gambling with their advertising clout. They "bet you can't eat just one".

There are over thirty thousand methods of weight control, from total fasting, to gastric stapling, yet 95% of these dieters will regain their weight within one year. You know it and I know it. DIETS DON'T WORK!! The Grapefruit Diet, the Zone Diet, the South Beach Diet, the High Fiber Diet, the Scarsdale Diet, the Beverly Hills Diet, and the Cambridge Diet have all been widely acclaimed. Even the Aitkin's Diet which advocates fasting and can actually be hazardous to your health will meet with some limited degree of success, but the key is limited. Dieting simply implies that you'll follow the program for a short time. You will go on a diet, and by the very definition, you will go off the diet. Alas, over an extended period of time, these "diets" are singularly unsuccessful at maintaining weight loss. So if you want to change your current weight, what do you need to do to succeed? Are you ready to stop riding the weight loss roller coaster? Are you ready to finally examine what you are doing and take your health seriously? If the answers to these questions are yes, then you have chosen the right book. The popularity of weight loss clinics, exercise salons, and health spas attest to the fact that we are spending billions of dollars a year to fight the Battle of the Bulge. But we're losing. Bound by fables, and hobbled by misinformation regarding diets, we flounder with the fragments of truth about weight loss, reduction and control. Now is the time to break away. Here, you are offered pair of Golden Slippers, and like Dorothy's magic slippers you have the power to go anywhere you want to and do anything you want to do, but here is the secret. You've got to THINK THAT YOU CAN. Like the little engine that thought he could, and like all the successful people who think they can, and DO, this program offers you the chance to break away. You are offered a method that can be followed easily no matter what you do and you will lose weight. The method is so simple, in fact that you will be tempted to say, "No". That won't work for me. I know that I can't do that and make it work. This method is a self styled plan, so you will individualize it for yourself and your lifestyle. This is not a one plan fits all method.

There is a clear process of change including decisional balancing, as you progress between the stages of change. There is what is termed the tyranny of the immediate priority of relationships. As you move through the stages of change you must understand the immediate priority of the relationship, understand the stages and your readiness to change and move through o allow you to progress through the stages. Directing change is client centered and involves change self talk. Using the ABC Model it involves the **A**ntecedents including all the emotions you need in place; empathy, discrepancy, and augmentation. **B**ehavior change begins with resistance and finally acceptance to the changing behavior. **C**onsequences involve understanding first, and then addressing the what, where and how. What will happen if, and then improving self efficacy based on the answers to the questions posed? The Tran theoretical model for change proposes that successful candidates must be psychologically ready to change. All individuals move through four phases of readiness when they begin a new weight management program. To find out your stage of readiness check the following stages and see which stage you fit into.

PRECONTEMPLATIVE STAGE: Ignorance is bliss. You are not ready to stop eating the foods that you like. You don't have time to increase your activity. Everyone in your family is "big". You don't see the point of losing weight. You have neither thought about, nor do you intend to lose weight within the next six months. You have not thought about what foods contribute to a problematic weight state. Neither do you believe that your weight is not a health issue, nor do you feel the need to take responsibility for your weight status or any changes within the next months. You do not feel that your health is affected by your weight. If asked, you do not intend to make any changes in your current intake pattern, and have little confidence that any weight management program will work for you. In fact, you may be convinced that you are not over fat, that everyone in your family is "big boned". Additionally, you frequently find yourself without a plan for meals either during the weekday or on weekends. If asked to rate your motivation to lose weight on a scale of 1-10, it would likely be less than three. I can understand why you feel that way. You are the adult and you are the one to decide when you are ready to lose weight. However, based upon my training and experience you are placing yourself at serious risk for heart disease, the development of diabetes and other weight related health risks. Even losing 10% of your current weight could be the most important thing that you can begin to think about today.

CONTEMPLATIVE STAGE: You have tried to lose weight before but… You want to know if I can give you a pill or if there is some food that will facilitate weight loss. You are thinking maybe your metabolism is to blame, or if you could only get back in shape and sit less often. I'm glad you are at least thinking about it. You are considering some change within the next six months. Currently, you are merely considering the possibility of weight loss. You are still not completely decided about making the decision to commit, and I can understand that. It's a life changing decision. You are an adult and you will know when the time is right for you to lose weight. You are willing to listen to reasons why you should consider changes at this time. It may be helpful to write down what one benefit of losing weight might be. Also jot down the reason why weight loss is not good for you at this time. Everyone who has ever lost weight has started here. At this point you have not made any changes in your activity, but you may have considered going to the gym, or thought about ways you might increase your activity, if this is what you have determined is wrong. You believe that if you just exercise at the gym, you can lose all the weight. In fact, you may just believe you are only out of shape, and if you start to exercise you will be back to your fit self again. You just need to take the time to exercise. However, at this time you are not convinced that you really should give this weight change any sort of priority. At this stage the tyranny of the immediate priority of relationships is evident. There is always something closer to the front burner on the stove that needs your attention more. You think it might be a good idea to do something about your current weight, but not before you take care of the immediate concerns of everyday life. You are not ready at this point to actively lose weight. If asked to rate your motivation to lose weight on a scale of 1-10, it would probably be 4-6. I am glad to see you are thinking about it. You are the adult here and it is totally up to you to know if this is right for you right now.

PREPARATION STAGE: You are tired of looking and feeling the way you do. You want to do something to start feeling better. You want to learn to eat healthier, and have even tried a low fat dressing which surprisingly was not horrid. You have decided to see if this may be something you could do. You are clear that the benefits of attempting to lose weight outweigh the negatives and you are making plans to start within the next thirty days. You have listened to the arguments that you should lose weight. This is likely provided by a health practitioner, and it may be prompted by a health issue that has been diagnosed, such as high blood pressure, high cholesterol, pre-diabetes, or diabetes. It's wonderful that you feel the decision to lose weight is important enough to think about right now. You may have started to take medication for a health concern and are planning to lose weight within the next thirty days. You are relating your need to change and checking your ability to make the necessary changes. You have decided that you are ready to start losing weight within the next thirty days with small changes. You have expressed a willingness to commit. You want to learn how to eat in a healthy manner, and you are starting to at least look at "diet" products in the store. If you have ever attempted to lose weight before you may want to review in your mind what worked for you in the past. Take time to analyze the previous roadblocks. In the past month you have been actively trying to increase your daily activity to keep from gaining any more weight, and on a scale of 1-10 you are at least at a 7-8 level to increase activity. You are not only focusing on what kind of activity to do you may have signed up at a gym, or a group support for weight management. Think about your social support system and identify the family members or friends who will support you as you begin to make this change. You do believe that your current weight may be an unhealthy weight. You will probably meet with success in any program that you begin.

ACTION STAGE: You are actively forming new habits. You are eating healthier and are surprised that the things you thought you would miss are not such a big deal. You are eating more vegetables and use fresh fruits to nibble when you want a snack. When you eat out, you split you meal with your partner, or just eat half and take a doggie bag home. Holidays may be a challenge but you are starting to manage with alternative plans. If you don't walk or do some sort of activity each day, you can tell the difference. You understand the difference between physical, emotional and situational hunger and are working to only eat when you are physically hungry. You have set up a number of achievable goals including the portion control of the foods you are eating. You have started an exercise or activity program and have increased your NEAT (**N**on **E**xercise **A**ctivities) daily. You have begun to form new habits. You have assessed the calories that you take in daily and have identified the discretionary Calories you do not need and will avoid. You may have decided to change from regular soda to water, and you are already experiencing weight loss either through your own efforts or through a structured program. You are actively changing behaviors. You are open to suggestions for diet and exercise changes. People have noticed that you have lost weight. You may need help in reviewing new skills or with the holiday meal plans. Motivation on a scale of 1 10 is generally 9-10 at this point. Additional dietary guidance and exercise changes will be effective for you now.

MAINTENANCE STAGE: You always get fresh fruits and vegetables and avoid snacking on candy or chips. When eating out you split the entrée. Restaurants serve meals that are just too big for one serving. Holidays and vacations are a challenge. You walk or use the NEAT pattern daily. You know that the time to eat is when you are physically hungry. You can change your mindset when you experience emotional or situational hunger. You have had a minimum of six months of effective weight loss. You have reached at least an intermediate goal and are actively attempting to maintain that loss. You are working to prevent a relapse. At this point, it is important to review what your initial weight was six months ago, and what your current weight is now. It is important to confirm that you have social and environmental support systems in place. At this time, you will need to reaffirm what you do on a routine basis regarding snacks, how you will handle holidays, and vacations. You will need to reassess your activity pattern to assure that it will support your routine intake to avoid weight regain. It's at this point that you will need to determine if you want to continue with your weight loss to another plateau, or if you are comfortable with your current status.

The choices within the plan can be made to fit into this program, and the correct choices will be what are right for you. This will work if you work from 9 to 5, whether you work the graveyard shift, or you don't work at all. You will gain confidence and skills, through practicing, and repeating, the simple steps. Do not limit yourself by saying that it won't work for you. It will. There will always be limits, but it's your choice to reach beyond your grasp. Go for the gusto. Go for the gold. This life's for you! Accept this plan and you can have that chocolate mousse. But remember, you must start today. If fact you have already started, by opening the cover of this book. In these next chapters you will be given the key to the city, the key to permanent weight control. You will begin to see your own personal motivations and your daily and weekly activity and intake patterns. You will increase your own personal health while learning weight control and the principles of nutrition that guide us in our information. **KNOWLEDGE IS POWER!** You will be given the key to permanent weight loss and control. You will see the habits that have developed the patterns causing weight gain, and you will be able to change those patterns if you want to. You will become slimmer, permanently. Now, you are invited to become an active participant, rather than a passive reader.

The book is divided into basic concepts and chapters. Work with the concepts in the chapters until you feel comfortable with and have mastered the principles. Only advance through the chapters at your own pace. Follow the format from the first, through the last chapter, rather than skipping ahead. This will insure that you build on the basic principles in the first chapters, and achieve results through personal change; change that you will be comfortable with. The results will be an invaluable arsenal for your own successful Battle against the Bulge. Now, with this book as your guide, you too can overcome your own mouth trap.

Although you may not realize it, the effects of stress, even positive stress upon your daily habits, and your food intake are undeniable. They affect what you are doing, even as you read this book, and the things that you will do in your lifetime. For example, if you're overweight, and want desperately to reduce, you will have a better rate of success if there are fewer upsetting experiences to contend with. That way you can focus on the one goal of weight loss. On the other hand, do you want to reduce but your spouse is out of work, or you just lost your job, the bank is about to foreclose on your mortgage, and you are ending an eight year affair with the mailman because he had his mail route changed, and the neighbors are threatening to sue you because your twelve year old son shot his air rifle through their bedroom window, and the ensuing commotion caused their pregnant, award winning Collie, to miscarry, then now may not be the time for any changes. Or perhaps the dealership where you just bought a lemon of a car left town under cover of darkness and now you have no recourse in recovering from the damages. Perhaps your husband just announced that he thinks that it might be a good time to retire. Or if your single daughter is pregnant, and is thirteen, I would probably not recommend this program now. You have too many other concerns. To check with your personal life situation, take the simple Stress Test Quotient Quiz that follows. And if the above description fits you, chin up, put the book on the shelf or offer it to the neighbor. Things will get better, but don't try to lose weight right now! To help you to control some of the stresses in your life, here are some tips to follow when you realize that you are in a stressful period.

Practice the best rest, eating and exercise patterns that you can manage. Just the simple act of getting eight hours of sleep a night will help to reduce the hormones that are triggered by stress. Eight hours of sleep will do several things. It will increase the adiponectin in your body. Adiponectin facilitates your body's ability to burn fat. It will also decrease gherin production. Gherin is the substance that will trigger the sensation of hunger in your body. Just body movement; frequently reduce the stresses you have been building. The simple act of shrugging your shoulders, rotating you head and breathing in deeply will relieve stress. During times of high stress you might want to consider avoiding caffeine during this time or at least decrease your intake of caffeine to less than 250 milligrams a day. These practices take a little time but will help to give you the feeling of more control and the realization that you are worth the effort. Good habits will add fuel to the fire that you've begun. When stress builds remember to stick to a schedule. Typically, stressful times are busy. Avoid getting overloaded. Make a list and delineate by level of importance. Delegate some responsibilities to others. This will motivate you to take action towards the solution, and help you to get a different prospective on the problem situation. Remember to try to prevent stress before it begins, but when it's too late...DON'T LET IT CONTROL YOU. Do something about it. Take a walk, listen to music, smile and find something to laugh about. Almost anything that you can think of is better than taking no action at all.

USE THE FOLLOWING TENSION RELEASE EXERCISES TO COPE WITH STRESS.

1. Head roll: Sitting relaxed, close your eyes, and roll your head clockwise. Stop, then repeat counter clockwise. Did you hear a creak? Good. It's that kind of tension that builds up to cause the little things to become unbearable.
2. Shoulder Shrugs: Sitting or standing, palms flat. Raise, and lower your shoulders. Repeat this ten times.
3. Shoulder Circles: Sitting or standing, palms flat, arms at side, roll shoulders forward then backward. Feel a stretch in your muscles, good. You're getting out the tension.

WHAT'S YOUR STRESS QUOTIENT?

Check those items that have happened to you within the past six months. It's more important how much has happened in a short period of time than how much has happened over your lifetime. Remember it wasn't the straw that broke the camel's back, it was the last straw.

CATEGORY I: ALLOW YOURSELF 2 POINTS FOR EACH ITEM CHECKED.TOTAL: _____

death of a spouse   relationship separation death/ family member
stopped smoking   personal injury/illness marriage loss of your job
martial reconciliation retirement   change family health
pregnancy   sexual difficulties   new family member

CATEGORY II: ALLOW 1 POINT FOR ITEMS IN THIS CATEGORY: TOTAL: _____

financial change   death of close friend
change in work   change work responsibilities
large mortgage on home   change in number of spousal arguments
foreclosure   child/sibling leaving home
in-law problems   revision of personal habits
problems at work

CATEGORY III: ALLOW 1/2 POINT FOR THESE. TOTAL: _____

Change in work habits   Change in work hours
change in school   change in residence
change in recreation   change social life
change in sleeping habits vacation
minor law violation

TOTAL POINTS SCORED FROM ALL CATEGORIES: TOTAL: _____

SCORE 30+ =   although you may want to lose weight, the present is definitely not the time. You have too much on your mind.
SCORE 20-29 = Work on reducing the irritants before reading further.

SCORE 10-19 = With a strong personality, you have a great probability for success, as long as less than half the points come from Category 1.

SCORE 10 or less indicates that there are relatively few stress situations time management skills that you know.

Break down the barriers that are keeping you from success today. Take care of the business that is the most pressing. When you reduce the irritants, you will then find it easier to reduce your adipose tissue. Your mental stability and health are as important to you as your physical health. In fact many would agree that the physical health hinges upon good mental health. To check your mental health and give yourself the greatest chance of success, take the time to analyze the results and rate your personal situation. Although you may not be able to change all the things that are causing you stress, if you change the things that you can change, you will be surprised that those problems that seemed insurmountable become less important. You will learn some things in your present situation that may surprise you. Then you will be better able to realize the importance needed to focus on your personal health and weight goals. You will begin to realize the importance that you must place on all phases of your life to make weight reduction and permanent weight control work for you. Don't let weight control take a back seat, make them a top priority. If negative thoughts keep you from acting, try the "Picture. Erase. Replace." technique to control your thoughts. Sit quietly and comfortably seated. Now force yourself to imagine an uncomfortable situation. Feel the feelings that come with the pictured situation and understand the feelings you are feeling. Now take the picture in your mind and frame it. Move it farther away from your vision. If you are in the picture, step out of it. Now make the picture darker and darker. Move it farther away from you, and begin to make the picture smaller and smaller. Make the picture smaller yet until it is the size of a postage stamp. Move it even farther from you. Now make the picture smaller and darker until it disappears. This has forced you to erase the situation that is negatively impacting you. Now bring the picture back. See if the feelings are less apparent. Repeat the above steps again until you notice a definite decrease in the emotional impact of this picture.

Now think of something pleasant. Notice your body position, and the feelings. Visualize the pleasant, restful feelings. Perhaps it is a picture of a picnic in the country or at the beach or any event where you are very much at ease. Now replace that with the picture that gave you discomfort. Repeat this until you have the pleasant comfortable feelings of control. Surround yourself with lighting, music and a seat that is comfortable. Take time for a short nap or bubble bath. Spend time doing something that will take your mind off the stressful situation. Read a pleasant book. Seek the company of a friend with an understanding ear. Many times problems can be minimized by simply talking them through. Take a physical break if possible, such as a vacation, or a simple change of scenery by changing rooms, taking a ride in the car train, or a walk. This is an example of gaining control in your environment.

HEALTH STYLE: SELF TEST

All of us want good health. Give yourself this health style self test and check the habits that you will want to concentrate on to increase your chances for success.

Do you avoid alcohol regularly?

Do you smoke cigarettes?

Do you eat a variety of foods daily including whole grains?

Fresh vegetables? Beans? Nuts and lean meats?

Do you limit fat and cholesterol from butter? Cream? Shortening?

Do you limit the amount of salt you eat?

Do you avoid too much sugar, sticky candy, and soft drinks?

Do you find it easy to express your feelings?

Do you have close friends and relatives to talk problems over with?

Do you get regular exercise daily?

Do you exercise to enhance muscle tone, and use part of leisure time to participate in family and individual activities?

If any of these questions left you squirming, then you're reading the right book. I will venture to say that 90% of you who answered honestly didn't answer the way you would have liked to answer these questions. DON'T DESPAIR! Remember, gradual change is the best anyway.

Never give up anything until you're ready to. There is no such thing as "SWALLOW IT WHOLE." Don't do it. You'll choke.

You don't *try* to do it. You do it, because you want to. One of the unfair consequences of overweight, or obesity is the terrible stigma that comes with being judged by society obsessed with thinness. Obesity is commonly assessed to be a result of laziness or lack of self control. The psychological burden that attitude imposes on someone who is overweight or obese can have far reaching effects on the overall mental health. If only society could "walk a mile" before they criticize. Think about the reasons you want to lose weight now. Is it because you feel uncomfortable, or is there medical pressure to reduce? Whatever the reasons, the most important and final reason must come from inside of you. That's the only way to become. Choose one of the answers on the list and change it, just for one day TODAY or in your own head. "Where there's a will, there's a way." Now, put those dreams into practice. Close your eyes, and think what you will look like when you have lost the weight that you're going to lose. Sit back, relax. Now sit up straight and proud. Dream those dreams. Think of the clothes that you will wear. Think where you will go. See yourself at some specific place. Listen to what other people are saying to you. Close your eyes and dream. Make your dream as real as you can make it. Our marvelous brain can work miracles. Visualization is powerful. Think of specific people, a special place, and even a particular conversation. Most of all see your success. If you cannot see this dream, don't go on until you do. This visualization is virtually tantamount to your success. If you truly want to lose weight, YOU CAN. But you have to think that you can. You have to see yourself doing it, before you even do it. You have to have a dream and dream that dream. Hold in your stomach. Sit up straight and proud. Close your eyes, and know that you can reach your dream. If you truly want to lose weight YOU CAN. Think about the reasons why you want to lose weight now. Is it because you feel uncomfortable? It has to be more than that. Is there medical pressure to reduce? Whatever the reasons, the final and most important reason must come from inside of you. The only way to participate is to make the reasons alive for you. Make the reasons, your reasons.

As a registered dietitian, while working at the Redondo Beach Medical Clinic, in Redondo, California my patients were usually referred by an endocrinologist, and were tasked with weight loss. Together, my patients and I set individual goals. A bar graph in the Torrance Boulevard office represented our visual goal. It represented what both I and my patients wanted. It was a living visual goal. In seven short months we collectively lost over four hundred pounds. You are encouraged to make a visual reminder. Write the date and the weight that you are today. Weigh at the same time of day. Weigh approximately three times weekly. Then as you trickle down you will see the results. These patients used a number of exercises to identify the external cues that signaled situational and emotional hunger; such as the sight of tasty h'or d'oeuvres at a party, or the clock on the wall "telling you that it's time for lunch". This is one of three types of hunger. The first, situational hunger may be especially true at work when you are involved in a mindless task or something that is boring or less than pleasant. At work, do you mindlessly go past the candy jar and grab one or more hard candies? An "externally controlled" person doesn't have an easy time keeping his or her weight controlled with huge amounts and a wide variety of tempting foods readily available unless you learn to identify this type of societally induced hunger as emotional or situational and then control the situation. Is there another way to bypass the desk with the candies? If not, can you look out the window at the wonderful skies and think about quitting time? Another example or situational hunger is when dining out. Restaurants offer a "16 ounce sirloin steak", which, by the way, provides more than the recommended daily intake of protein for a 246 pound individual. Buffets and salad bars urge patrons to have "all you can eat" for one set price. Many people are convinced that it's okay to gorge themselves here because it would be a "waste" or a "shame" to pass up such a good deal. The situation can be controlled. Order what you want, and ask for a doggie bag. That will provide you with a second meal out, tomorrow without the calorie consequences.

"Eating makes me feel better." Emotional hunger may cause some individuals to use food as a pacifier when you're upset or nervous. In fact, it may go all the way back to your childhood and the way you were comforted as a child. Food is a symbol of love. During childhood we may have been given a lollipop for being "good." Birthdays were filled with cake and ice cream. During our infancy these associations made us see food as an expression of our love. Knowing the reasons for our feelings is half the battle. We have become programmed by these habits, sights, smells and all the other environmental and emotional stimuli. Once we have identified these feelings and their roots, we can begin to break the chain.

Now write five reasons for wanting to change your body image.

1._____
2._____
3._____
4._____
5._____

Are these your own personal reasons for wanting to change your own body image permanently? If you answered yes, congratulations, you will succeed...If not...think again. They must be your OWN reasons for wanting to be slim. Two persons out of three are overweight or obese. Statistics tell us that the number of deaths and diseases related to obesity climbs yearly. In this world of societal evils of fast foods, sumptuous gourmet meals, and the three martini lunch, obesity takes its toll, coupled with hypertension, diabetes, and heart disease. The number one killer, heart disease is intimately linked to obesity. It's no secret. We, Americans, are surely eating ourselves into an early grave. But what are we to do? Give up every delicacy? Every sweet morsel of food? Go to a health store and pay outrageous prices for 'organic" foods, or an "assurance" of quality or wholesomeness? Never again sample an Italian pastry? Never again taste a bit of "je ne sait quoi?' NONSENSE! What we must do is learn to eat sensibly today. When we have accomplished this, we can eat anything that we want. Notice that the word is ANYTHING not as MUCH AS. The first key to sensible eating is control of our portion size. If you usually eat two, have one. If you drink a large, drink a medium or a small. If you order a super sized, usually, you are super sizing yourself as well. Order a small. You're the person who can exert control, and you can learn to become slim by controlling your portion sizes. If you use two dips of salad dressing, use one. The food will still taste good. In fact, it may taste better when you begin to eat sensitively.

Ralph Waldo Emerson is quoted as saying, "Enthusiasm is one of the most powerful engines of success. When you do a thing, do it with all your might. Put your whole soul into it. Stamp it with your own personality. Be active. Be energetic. Be enthusiastic and faithful and you will accomplish your objective. Nothing great was ever accomplished without enthusiasm." Remember, when you take on this great challenge that you are about to succeed at...Do exactly that. When you find a form of exercise that you enjoy, do it with enthusiasm. Take up Zumba. Begin to learn how to roller skate. If you think that this is just another ho-hum "cure-all", you need to rethink your mind set. Your mind is a marvelous computer, and what thoughts you feed it, will be fed right back to you. The most powerful resource that you possess is your mind. Remember, whether you think that you can or you can't accomplish something...you're right!

Patience and determination are two of the blueprints to success in weight management, and control. So, for your health and well-being, be patient and allow yourself to become the lean person you are within. You must admit to yourself that it won't happen tomorrow. But it can begin to happen today. You didn't wake up one morning fat! Incorporate new habits which can remain throughout your life. Make a goal that you can reach easily. One of the most difficult things that I teach my clients to do is set goals that they can reach. When I ask my new clients what they want to accomplish, what their goal is; inevitably they say; "I want to lose 100 pounds" "I want to lose 50 pounds." "I want to lose 25 pounds." That's a lot to expect of any one person all at once. The sky might fall tomorrow. What do you want to accomplish today?

Successful weight loss needs to be redefined. What if you weigh 300 pounds? Your goal shouldn't be to get down to what society has determined to be your "ideal weight". Think yourself thin realistically. Lose ten per cent of your current weight within six months. If that weight loss meant months upon months of endless deprivation, denial of gourmet foods, birthday parties, and anniversary treats, avoidance of every perceivable food related "reward" imaginable...I wouldn't do it, would you? Instead I would put that information into my computer brain, and the answer I wanted, I would get. "It's not worth all the pain. I like myself better this way. My whole family has "big bones". I'm not that fat."

It's the same thing as taking someone to a huge estate and telling them that their job should be to clean up all the grounds of this estate with acres and acres of debris. That is their goal. What's more the grounds have not been maintained. There are weeds growing everywhere and the entire property is in a horrible state of disrepair. Or someone leads you to the inside of this enormous palatial home, that hasn't seen the other side of a broom, or mop for eons, and tells you that your goal is to make that property sparkle. Yuck! I don't know about you, but my first impression would be to walk over the horizon and see if I could get a better offer for work! Maybe that's why the bear went over the mountain! But that's exactly what you do when you set an unrealistic goal! You provide yourself with a formidable task, and believe me when I say that your marvelous computer mind will find ways to help you overcome this "problem".

Set small goals, goals that you can't help achieving. It can be as simple as substituting fruit as a snack for Doritos. If you watch TV or read, don't eat while doing those activities. When you eat, only eat. One of my clients was very successful in her profession, but she insisted that she was not successful in reducing, yet she sat with me and in conversation, told me of losing 70 pounds, at one particular time and then fifty at another time and ninety at another time. She had failed to see that every time she set a goal, she reached it. The problem was that once she had reached her goal she didn't set another goal to maintain that weight for the next day, or week or month. She had reached her goal. Be very careful not to let that happen to you. Your goal once that you've reached a weight that you find desirable should include all the things that you did to lose the weight in the first place. Then set another goal. Always be setting goals. You've probably heard that the exciting part about a goal is not the goal itself, but getting there. This client had proved it in spades! An excellent book on goal setting is "Targets" By Leon Tec, M.D... It's how to set goals for yourself and reach them.

Now, let's go back to the palatial home, on the debris laden estate. What if someone told you your goal was to wash one small window, or one tile on the floor? Or to pick up one piece of paper or weed one small section of the royal garden? And when you had finished, you were applauded?? Would you want to do one small window, or one more tile, or one more small section of the royal garden??? That works! You don't even have to ask for applause outside yourself. When you accomplish a task, the fact you have set the goal and achieved it is enough. In fact in many instances, the job well done will be excellent reinforcement, the five pounds, or the three pounds, or the one pound lost will be reward in itself. If you don't get the feedback that you think that you deserve, create your own positive feedback. Remember, it is you that you are trying to impress.

Lose only five pounds at a time. Make your goal the 300 mark then the 295 mark then the 290 mark. Applaud yourself mentally when you reach your goals. Then, most importantly, **SET NEW GOALS**. Another of my clients related a story that was very sad. She was going to Weight Watchers, and being successful then she made the mistake of telling some people that she had lost a certain number of pounds. As she continued to be successful, she developed a cheering section at her workplace.

"You want everyone to know how much you lost, but you don't necessarily want anyone to know how much that you weighed." She intimated.

Although she was very successful at her weight loss, the cheering section backfired. She began hiding the actual number of pounds that she lost from her associates, because they were adding the lost pounds up even more accurately than she was. Dr. Blackburn (Top Clin.Nutr.2 (2), 1987) proposed that the primary goal for any single course of weight loss should be based not on standard height-weight tables but rather on a 10-15% loss of your usual body weight over a six month period. There were undeniable influences and every best intention may be thwarted if the timing or the environment is not right. This is a world of societal evils, sumptuous gourmet foods, and endless snacks. But you can break the cycle of your own health destruction. Follow the chapter format from the first through the last. This will ensure that you are building the basic principles in the first chapters to achieve the personal change that you will be comfortable with. The results will be an invaluable arsenal for your own successful battle against the bulge. When you have accomplished this, you can eat anything you want, not "as much as". A major premise of sensible eating is portion size. If you usually have two…have one. If you drink an extra large…Drink a medium. If you order a large, order a small. You are choosing to minimize your needs, and you are the person with the control. You are the customer and the customer is always right. When you exert that control with portion sizes you can become slim as you minimize your portion size. If you use two scoops of salad dressing on your salad, use one. The food will still taste good; in fact it may taste better.

Think back to the last diet that you followed. Something motivated you to pick up that diet book. Something motivated you to begin to watch what you were eating and something motivated you to begin to look at the foods you ate in a day. Success comes in many forms. No matter the shape, size or age you are in you can be successful. Success means achieving the right weight for you. It means taking a long look at yourself honestly and then taking steps to make the improvements that will help you for long term success. Success means taking one day at a time and beginning to feel good about you from the inside out.

Are you are interested in losing weight for the summer to be able to fit into that bathing suit or for next week to fit into the dress or pair of slacks that have been hanging in the closet? Is it because the doctor advised you to lose some weight for your own health benefit? It is you who must take the first very important step in exerting control in your present environment.

Sit down and take stock of yourself and your situation. Think about the quality of your life and your health. One of the consequences of obesity is the terrible stigma that comes from being judged for your appearance by a society obsessed with thinness. Obesity historically has commonly been assessed to be a result of laziness and a lack of self-control. The psychological burden that attitude imposes on someone who is overweight can have far reaching effects on your overall mental well being. But the most important of all should be the driving urge to become healthy. You only have one body. If you get sick, where are you going to live? Think about the reasons why you want to lose weight now. Is it because you feel uncomfortable? It has to be more than that. Is there medical pressure to reduce? Whatever the reasons, the final and most important reason must come from inside of you. This process will require your participation. The best way to participate is to make the reasons alive for you, not because your mother-in-law wants you to lose weight. The goal you want should be a living visual goal. Now, its time to make those dreams your reality. Pick up your pencil and write your goal, for yourself alone. Be honest. This is your goal. You are about to make your dream a reality.

I,_____want to lose weight because
_____. Think about what you think you look like now. I don't mean what someone else thinks you look like. What do *you think you look like?* Do you think that you can lose weight? Or are you

still giving yourself the excuses that "all my family is big boned"? I just can't lose weight. I haven't been that weight since I was in college, or since I was in the military. I have a lot of muscle. If I lose weight I will die. If I get lower than___ number of pounds I don't look good. Let me remind you of the most important secret. If you think you can...YOU CAN! If you don't think you can, you're right too. You can become what you want to become in terms of the weight you want to be. Have you ever listened to the lyrics in a song by Neil Diamond? "Have you heard about the frog that dreamed about becoming a prince…and then became one?" "Though the scenes and the names have changed, my story's the same one." Listen to the lyrics you sing to yourself inside your head. They will dictate what you think you can and what you think you can't do. If you think you can, you will. Where there's a will, there's a way. "If ye have faith of a grain of mustard seed … nothing will be impossible unto you".

Sit back and relax. Close your eyes and think about what you will look like when you have lost the weight that you are going to lose. Think of the clothes you will wear. Think of where you will go. See yourself in some specific spot. Paint the picture in your mind's eye as realistically as possible. Think of the outfit you will be wearing, the shoes you will have on. Make your dream as real as you can make it. Think of specific people and even a specific conversation. Most of all see your success. If you truly want to lose weight, you can. However, you have to see yourself doing it, even before you do it. You have to think you can. You have to have a dream of success. Hold in your stomach. Sit up straight and proud. Close your eyes and know that you can reach your dream. Make the dream your reality. If you truly want to lose weight and reach your healthy weight goal, you can.

Make your dreams real. Why do you believe you are overweight now? If you thought about stress, or the work environment, the next set of exercises may help to change your mind set. Very simply, balance the imbalance in the energy equation of your body by controlled eating. If you eat more Calories than you use, you will gain weight. If you eat fewer Calories than you use, you will lose weight. There is no mumbo jumbo. There are no magic combinations, and there are no special combinations of Calories that will magically make the pounds disappear. Our systems have become confused in our society, where the food companies are in a very sophisticated and highly competitive race to sell you their food.

Advertising brings food to our attention. New products virtually unknown on the market can become an overnight success with advertising. Food companies influence our choices in countless blunt and subtle ways. It is difficult to measure the influence of their advertisements in our food choices but it is inexplicably intertwined. Food advertising encourages overeating. It directs weight conscious consumers to purchase special "diet" foods that are more expensive and unnecessary. Colorful and beautifully photographed food advertisements create a desire for the products and its constant media exposure in magazines, newspaper and supermarket advertisements, television and the Internet. America is the breadbasket of the world and the large food corporations who engage in the process of selling their products are no better than the proverbial used car salesman. They will sell anything and anyway they can. The only difference is the fact that these companies invest billions of dollars in market research and advertising to ensure they get their fair market share of your dollars. If you think these companies care whether a certain product can lower your cholesterol, or another product will help you lose inches from your waist, you are dead wrong. They want to create a product that looks and sounds too good to resist. What these companies care about is their bottom line and the dollars they may be able to extract from your wallet with their intriguing advertising slogans.

The problems of overeating are complex. Research indicates that if you are overweight you are more likely than a normal weight person to eat for reasons that are not considered true physiological hunger. Instead you may be more motivated by such external cues as the sight of a food commercial advertising some delicious looking, if truly unhealthful morsel. The next time you are watching television and a food commercial is shown, watch your reaction. Or when you go to the movies, watch what happens to many of the people in the theater audience, when the advertisement for their fat ridden popcorn flashes on the screen. Even the clock on the wall, especially if you are at work, bored or doing some less than pleasant task, may be enough for you to think about food. That is not hunger. That is boredom. Your internal clock is telling you its time for "lunch" and a wonderful excuse to stop doing a mindless task. I don't have to tell you that if you are externally controlled you need to be conscious of wanting to eat for emotional or situational reasons. We want to eat because of physical hunger. If you are lured by cues in the environment you will need to reprogram you mind to keep your weight in check. There are a wide variety of delectable foods readily available to tempt us. Restaurants from fast food to fine dining have all joined the super size revolution. Restaurants offering a sixteen-ounce sirloin are providing you with 975 Calories, 45 grams of total fat and 112 grams of protein. That one serving of steak provides the RDI (Recommended Daily Intake) of protein for a two hundred and fifty pound person. It provides twice the RDI for cholesterol for any person and nearly half of the Calories needed in an entire day. Fast food restaurants are past masters of the Super Size Revolution. Buffets and salad bars urge patrons to have "all you can eat" for one set price. Sadly we have been convinced that its "okay" to gorge ourselves in such places because is would be a waste of time or a shame to pass up such a great deal. How many times have you eaten dessert not because you were still hungry, but because it "came with the meal" or it just looked too good to say no?

"Eating makes me feel better." The role of food in our social life may be a contributing factor to over eating and overweight. We comfort our friends with candy and fruit. We thank our hostess with a box of sweets or a bottle of wine. We welcome guests with a tasteful dinner that may be too high in Calories, sauces and then even add the inevitable dessert. We exchange recipes and compliment the cook of a special dish without even researching the Calorie, or fat or carbohydrate content of the food. Emotional reasons may cause you to use food as a pacifier especially when you are upset, or nervous. In fact, those feelings may be seeded in our childhood and the way we were comforted as a child. During childhood, we may have been given a lollipop or an ice cream bar or a cookie for being a good little boy or girl. Birthdays were filled with cake and ice cream. It was initially during our infancy, that these associations were made. Food became a symbol of love. Almost everyone has a group of traditional customs. Do you cook greens with bacon fat or use sour cream on blintzes or baked potatoes. These are high fat habits. Food habits are the sum of many experiences with food. To some people, wasting food is considered sinful. To others food has been used as reward foods to lure a child to eat. "If you don't eat your vegetables, you can't have dessert." The "clean plate club" has been highly overrated. You won't help the people who are starving in the world by eating when you are not hungry. If you have been exposed to these pressures when you were growing up, significant others in your life have encouraged a distorted view of the place food should have in your life. You will only succeed in adding excess burden to your own physique. To some parents, a fat child is a healthy child. This couldn't be farther from the truth. In fact, lean people live longer than their overweight or obese counterparts.

Knowing the reasons for our feelings is half the battle. We have become programmed by these behaviors. They are deeply seeded behaviors, and habits. The sight and smell or food in the environment can be the stimulus for us to want that food to recapture that feeling, and feel loved at a time when things are not going as well as we had hoped. Patience and determination are two of the blueprints to success in weight management and lifetime control. For your health and well being be patient and allow yourself to become lean at your own pace. You must realize that it will not happen tomorrow. But it can begin today. You didn't wake up one morning fat! If you think back you can track your pattern of weight gain throughout your life. Additionally, there is usually a defining moment in life when you gained a portion of your weight, but after the event, you did not go back to your previous set weight. Think about the life defining moments, and the stressors that you endured. Was it a wedding, a divorce, the birth of a child, the death of a parent? It was probably a stressful time in your life. Both good stressors and bad stressors can affect you. When we have identified these as invalid reasons for wanting to eat, the next step will be to break the chain.

Habits are changeable because they are learned behaviors. Pavlov's dog salivated when the bell rang. That is a learned response. We too are conditioned by our environment and everything not the least of which are the clock, the billboards, and the commercials. The advertising companies know this well and use it expertly in their advertising schemes to sell their products in this highly competitive market.

You can change your response by avoiding or reassigning the cues. Drive home an alternate way to avoid the convenience store or the bakery. Look past the billboard that tells you the "burgers are better" and avoid the temptations. Don't confront yourself with them. Use the same psychology that you use with your children, because after all it may well be the child in you that is demanding the "instant gratification". If your children want to go swimming and you have firmly told them "no", do you then drive them to the lake so they can see the crystal blue water and feel the cooling breeze? Of course you don't you distract them with other things. Don't you have something better to do than eat when you aren't hungry?

Chapter 2

Direct Yourself to Win
The Power of Visualization and Goal Setting

Goal setting is easy, right? You simply decide what is it you want to do, and then you set out to do it. If it's so simple, why do so many things that we want to do not get done? Why, then if these are things we REALLY want to do, and are important to us, do the days slip by without us completing those tasks that will take us closer to our goals? All of us have set goals for ourselves, whether in work, or in relationships with others, to improve ourselves in our careers, or to learn to interact ore effectively with out children. Yet for any number of reasons, we never accomplish our goals. We explain,

"I'm just too busy."

"I'm not really that much overweight."

"I am just big boned."

The first key is know what you want to do. Again, the key is **want to**. When I ask my patients what goal they want to accomplish, they inevitably say,

"I need to lose some weight." Exactly how much weight they intend to lose is frequently unclear, but one thing is certain. The goal is often lofty! 25, 50 or 100 pounds. That's a lot to expect of any one person all at once. The sky might fall tomorrow. What do you want to accomplish today?

Weight loss is directly related to the degree of interest or enthusiasm a person has about losing weight. As interest and enthusiasm wanes, the weight loss slows down. The greater your determination to lose weight, the more lasting your weight loss will be. Since that is proven, it becomes more important for you to understand that enthusiasm is one of the principles of permanent weight loss.

You've undoubtedly learned through various sources that the successful weight loss program includes a Calorie controlled diet, with increased and sustained routine exercise. Many people additionally resort to pharmacological appetite suppressants, or diet pills. Although diet, exercise and appetite suppressants, properly applied will cause some degree of success the success is limited. Usually, patients regain the weight that was lost, and gradually resume their original eating habits. There is a missing ingredient and it includes the most powerful organ in your body. Your brain! You can substitute good habits for faulty habits. Those faulty habits are the ones that allowed you to eat too much and burn up too few Calories. Modifying your habits is a very important part of the answer. It includes not only knowing but modifying the speed at which you eat, knowing where you eat, and under what circumstances. It may include altering you lifestyle, substituting activities for eating or changing from activities that center around food. It involves changing your attitude, setting realistic goals, and learning to cope with stresses and situations that may sabotage your reducing efforts.

Successful weight loss should be redefined. If you weigh three hundred pounds, then your goal should not be to get down to what society has determined to be "your ideal weight". The first goal must be a manageable and obtainable goal. Your attitude, or mind set is the rose colored glasses through which you perceive your world. You use this attitude to filter and imprint events. This serves as your screen to protect your inner most feelings and fears. If your attitude is a winning attitude, you will be less scarred by failure and defeat. Did you know that Edison was never defeated, although his teachers told him he was "too stupid to learn anything"? And when questioned about the fact that he failed to make a light bulb 1,000 times before he succeeded, he argued. I didn't fail one thousand times. The light bulb was an invention that took one thousand steps. The process of inventing a light bulb was an inventive process of one thousand steps just as inventive attitude spells success. A defeatist attitude produces a self defeating circle. You begin to feel guilt and self hate then self pity and less than desirable behaviors. The promise that you can eat all the foods that are "bad" for you and still lose weight is what we want to hear. How many of the advertisements for weight loss plans proclaim. You can eat anything you want? How about the ad that exclaims,

"I can eat chocolate every day!"

That is in fact, the basis behind many fad diets. Instead of setting realistic goals, we put the erroneous information into our computer brains and the answer we want, we will get."

It's not worth the pain."

I like myself better this way."

"I could never lose weight and get down to that number."

"I'm not really fat. I'm big boned."

"My whole family is big. I've always been heavy."

"I just can't lose weight."

"If I lose weight I will die."

"If I get lower than_____pounds, I don't look good."

These statements reflect an internal loss of control over events in your world. I have news for you. Genetics do determine your bodies build which does influence your weight, since frame reflects the chest size and hip width as well as bone density and size. If you have a large frame your ideal weight may be higher. But, your whole family may be "big" because of the eating habits that the entire family has been following for years. At the time you were growing up you may not have had any control, but as an adult you do now! You can take control and you can make it happen. It's time to stop blaming and complaining. The time to act is now. Do you really think that you can lose weight? Really? Let me tell you a little secret. If you think you can, you can! If you don't think you can. You are right too! You can become what you want to become. Remember the lyrics in a Neil Diamond song?

"Have you heard about the frog that dreamed about becoming a prince...and then became one? Well, though the scenes and the names have changed, my story's the same one." Replay those lyrics whether as a song or in your own head. They will dictate to you that you can do it. Remember the mustard seed, and where there is a will, there's a way. Now, put those dreams firmly in your mind. Close your eyes, and think what you will look like when you have lost the weight that you plan to lose. Sit back and relax. What will you are wearing? Where will you go? Dream again about a specific place, and specific time. Imagine the people who will be with you. Listen to the conversation. Make this as real as possible. Make this commitment for you. Make the reasons alive for you, not for your mother or your mother-in-law. The goal you want should be a living visual goal. Now, transform those dreams into a living goal. Write your goals down.

'Oh, it's not such a big goal." You might say.

"It's not important enough to write down."

"It takes too much time."

"I don't have a pen."

"I can do it without writing it down."

Increase the value of your life by placing value on the things you really want. If the goal has value, then it is worth the effort. You alone must take the responsibility to do it. Let me remind you of secret you already know. If you don't write it down, it's not a concrete goal. It's a simple daydream, a good intention.

I,_____will lose weight because_____.

I want to lose _____pounds. I know I will achieve this goal.

Signed: _____Date: _____

Very simply balance and imbalance in the energy equation will cause weight loss or weight gain. If you eat more Calories than you use, you will gain weight. If you eat fewer Calories than you use, you will lose weight. Changing behaviors is not necessarily easy. It involves compromise and decisions that are sometimes difficult to make. The entire process is emotion filled, and it requires physical, mental and emotional commitment. Imagine that huge estate that has been neglected for years. The grounds are littered with debris, and overgrown with weeds everywhere. Inside this palatial home hasn't seen the other side of a broom or mop for years. It is your goal to clean the property inside and out and restore it to its former glory days. I don't know about you but my first impression would be to walk over the horizon and see what was behind door Number Two. That is exactly what you are doing to yourself when you set an unrealistic goal. You provide yourself a formidable task, and believe me when I tell you that your marvelous computer brain will find ways to help you overcome this problem.

Instead, set small goals that are easily achievable. It can be a simple as substituting fruit for a snack of Doritos. It could be to change one small habit, for example, when you eat, only eat. That means if you watch television, don't snack. When you read, don't snack. When you eat, only eat. Choose one place to eat in your home. It can be the dining room table, but eat all meals, and snacks at this place. Be certain it is a comfortable and attractive place. If you eat in different places throughout the home, you will find increasingly different things stimulate you to want to eat. Your environment for eating will improve as you become more aware of the act of eating and the stimuli that contribute to overeating.

The exciting part about goal setting is not the goal itself, but getting there. It's the journey not the destination. Reward yourself for losing weight. Choose a reward that you really like other than food. Eating has, for many people become a reward. By giving yourself something you'd really like to have, you can help change your eating behavior. You might decide to give yourself $5.00 for every pound you lose. Decide what you are going to do with the money before hand. Use the money to take a trip or do something you really want to do.

Now, going back to the debris-laden estate, what if someone told you that your goal was not to clean the whole estate, but merely to pickup, one piece of litter, or wash one small windowpane and you would be rewarded. That makes all the difference. That is attainable. You would be more apt to do that. In fact, you might even consider doing it without reward, because the job well done is often reinforcement enough. Now apply that same principle to food. Eat when you are hungry not when you are bored. Set a realistic weight goal you can attain. Lose only one pound at a time. Make your goal 299 pounds.

However, be certain you give that pound enough significance. It takes 3,500 Calories to make one pound of fat. Then to lose one pound of fat, you will have to burn up or avoid 3,500 Calories in one week. If you break it down further, that means you would need to cut out 500 Calories from your meal intake every day! That's a lot!. One of my patients was very successful in her profession, but insisted she could not lose weight. Yet in conversation she told me about losing seventy pounds, at one time in her life, and of fifty another, and ninety pounds yet another. What she failed to see was that every time she set a goal for herself, she would reach it. The problem was that once she attained her goal for some specific event, she would then go back to her old habits, and inevitably regain the weight. Unfortunately, when we regain weight, what frequently happens is the rebound effect. You will regain the weight originally lost, and gain some additional weight over what you had been before. Applaud yourself mentally when you attain that goal. Then and most importantly, set a new goal for one pounds less. Aim for 298 pounds. You can get there. Then do it again. Further, don't let the weight be the goal. Make the healthy eating habits you have acquired be the goal.

If you set your goal to lose only one pound in a week, and continued to follow the one pound a week rule and keep it off, you will have lost 52 pounds in a year. The trick is to keep it off, so you want to be sure that those pounds are gone forever by changing your daily eating habits and activity patterns. Change your daily schedule to be certain that the time you want to eat is not a conditioned response. Many times we crave food at a particular time especially if the task we are doing is not challenging or boring. If you are used to coming home to a cocktail and snacks, stop the snacking. You are reinforcing your arrival home with the eating reflex. Don't substitute a low Calorie snack. That will encourage snacking. Even modest weight loss results in reducing physiologic stress by improving heart function, blood pressure, glucose tolerance, sleep disorders, respiratory function, and allows, in many cases, for a decrease in some medications associated with the above conditions. This improved health will often be reinforcement itself and minimizes the redounding weight.

Doctor Blackburn proposed that the primary goal for any single course of weight loss should not be based on standard height-weight tables, but on a goal of 10% of your current body weight over a certain period of time. Clinical Nutrition (1987). This may not sound like a lofty goal, but it is realistic and this is important to making a goal attainable. Take the weight loss in steps, rather than going down a slide. You may say,

"The slide is faster. I want to lose this weight by next week." The problem with the slide is that is the beginning of a weight loss roller coaster. Goals must be realistic. You cannot expect to lose ten pounds in one week, no matter what the miracle weight loss clinic are saying today. If you have a rapid weight loss, it is usually because of a lack of adequate fluid intake. That can cause another whole set of problems. Your goal should be fat weight loss not water loss. You want to lose weight for yourself, to satisfy yourself.

One of my clients related a story that should be a lesson to all who want to let everyone know that they are losing weight. She was going to Weight Watchers and was successfully losing a significant amount of weight. As her success became apparent she made the mistake of telling some people that she had lost a certain number of pounds. As her success continued, she developed a cheering section at work. However, sadly, her cheering section backfired. She confided,

"You want everyone to know how much weight you've lost, but you don't necessarily want anyone to know how much you weighed." She began to hide the actual number of pounds that she had lost, because her work mates were more accurate at adding up the pounds than she was.

Trickle down, and when you reach your goal, maintain the habits that helped you meet your target weight. Say, "No" to the habits that are destroying your self-esteem. You remember you can do it if you think you can. You will begin to think you can, just by saying,

"I can do it. I know I can lose weight." Follow the advice that is outlined in this book, and do go slowly. Go chapter by chapter until you have mastered the techniques in each of the chapters. Use close weight monitors. You can give yourself positive reinforcement for the many changes you are making in the types of foods that you consume in a day. Particularly with weight reduction, the importance of weight loss results cannot be overstressed. If there is only one indicator of weight loss and that is the scales, then the accomplishment of eating 3,500 Calories less than you need somehow isn't gratifying enough. This is particularly true when the scale seems "stuck" no matter how much you watch your intake or high fat, high Calorie, or high simple carbohydrate foods, or how much you increase your exercise. Remember that the regulation of weight is probably over a weekly rather than a daily period. Daily fluctuations are probably fluid related. So, let's work on specific goals and use the change in the scales weekly, as an affirmation that you are doing the right thing. That having been said, it is imperative that you do use a scale. Weigh yourself weekly, and record the results. If you hit one of the speed bumps, it's easier to get back on track and re-lose two pounds rather than wait for the semi-annual trip to the physician's office, and realize you have gained another ten pounds that you will have to lose.

Goal setting gets you on the right track, and thinking the right thoughts keeps you there. You can do it if you think that you can. One of the most important aspects of permanent weight loss is you positive cognitive ecology. Positive thoughts bring a positive attitude, along with its benefits and advantages. Negative thoughts will never allow you to gain the full control that you need to bring about permanent positive changes. The following statements can help you gain positive control in your everyday thoughts and actions.

Overeating will not be rewarded or punished.

I will be very selective in the foods I choose to eat.

I will choose the healthful foods that will bring me the most positive benefits.

I will be aware of all of the foods I eat.

I will learn to choose the less harmful of two junk foods.

I will learn to choose the most healthful and satisfying foods for me.

I will lose weight to satisfy myself.

I will take one day at a time, one meal at a time, and one situation at a time.

If I am not watching my intake well one day, it destroys nothing.

Everyday is a new day.

Success in losing weight permanently will be more likely to occur in an environment of positive thoughts. You have the ability to create that environment. Today is a perfect day to start developing your own positive cognitive ecology. You are responsible for your actions and the past will only help if you can learn from the mistakes that you have made. Think about it. Many people, in an attempt to be perfect make excuses for not taking responsibility for their actions. We all get to make the final choice.

"If I hadn't gone on that cruise, I wouldn't have gained that extra ten pounds." You alone have the ultimate control over your situation. The extra weight you want to lose didn't magically appear overnight. It didn't appear the day you left the service, the day you disembarked from the cruise liner, or the day you changed jobs. You gained that extra weight during the nine months of pregnancy that extra 10, or 20 or more pounds but it didn't disappear when the baby was born. You gained weight slowly, day by day. Those 10 pounds are equivalent to 35,000 extra Calories or an average of four thousand extra Calories each month. That's just fewer than 1000 extra Calories a week or less than 143 extra Calories each day. That's equal to two extra glasses of wine, or one 12 ounce Cola or other soft drink. It's about 20 potato chips, or a handful of nuts, or one ounce of American cheese. For every extra 3,500 Calories that you ate, your body had the ability to save those extra Calories in case you needed them later. Your body puts them into temporary storage as glycogen. When your body didn't need those extra Calories in the temporary storage bin, you body wisely put them into long term storage as adipose tissue, in case of a famine. In America, the bread basket of the world, that famine never came.

Unfortunately, you became less active, so you used fewer Calories. You became older and your basal metabolic rate, the energy you need to run all the organs in your body slowed as you aged. When the glycogen wasn't needed, your body found a long-term storage for that energy in case you needed it in the future and those 3,500 Calories was converted to adipose tissue, and one extra pound of fat appeared. What's more, your body regulates metabolism and Calorie and energy management on a weekly rather than a daily basis. It's like putting money in a bank. Your body's metabolism is more like a budget. If you need more than you use during the day, your body is able to call upon the extra stores, much like a savings bank. If we, individuals could save our money as well as we save our Calories we would be far richer society than we are today.

The reverse is also true. You can eat 500 less Calories than you need, and in seven short days, you can reverse the storage process, and lose one pound of fat. Eat only as much as you need. Eat when you are hungry and stop when you are full. Use your fat stores and save your money, what a concept. You only need to know what your budget is and this procedure will work for you.

You must realize that all the diets in the world will not work unless you control your mental attitude towards food. The way to succeed is to get your positive mental attitude in gear and avoid the problems that get you sidetracked. That's easy to say, right? Decide what it is that you need, then get the things done that will lead you closer to that goal. Know what will satisfy you. In the world today, and ten years from now, we will continue to face multitudinous stresses daily. The key is not to let the little things get you down. If your balancing your checkbook and your pen runs out of ink, do you stop? You simply delay your task while you find another pen and then return to your task, right? You overcome that obstacle and accomplished the goal.

Sadly, too many people become discouraged by a temporary set back. If you are following weight conscious principles and because of an unavoidable change of plans, you find yourself invited to share pizza with friends instead of eating your brown bag lunch at work, it's a temptation for a high fat, high Calorie meal that you can use to your advantage. It's not the end of the world but it is the end of many a diet. Then the excuses begin.

"Oh, I was bad." "I really blew it." Then the guilt begins.

"I'm no good anyway." "I'll never do this."

"I just can't control myself." **STOP** right there! Think about the pen that ran out of ink. That's life. You can shift into second gear just as easily as you can shift into reverse. Having that piece of pizza may not be the best choice but if you know what you are agreeing to you can redefine your budget for the rest of the day. One piece of Toni's Sausage and Pepperoni Pizza with Italian style pastry crust (147 grams) is about434 Calories and about 23 grams of fat. But if you know that and you goal for the day of avoiding 500 Calories, then you can either have a half a slice and a large salad with vinegar, or decide to increase your exercise to burn those extra Calories instead! What ever you do, don't degrade yourself. You've lost one or five or twenty-five pounds, and that's something you can be proud of.

You decide what it is you will do to attain your final objective. What will give you the most satisfaction? What is it that you need? Then, when you hit those inevitable set backs, those depressing speed bumps, those "Oh, I've just got to have a candy bar days" think of that pen that ran out of ink. It's only a speed bump and certainly not the obstacle that is going to stop you from reaching the most important goal you have ever set for yourself. Your goal of good health!

Once you have identified that, then negotiate those Calories and fat in that candy bar. One Mounds candy bar (about 1.9 ounces) has 258 Calories and 14 grams of fat. But one snack size Mounds (about 19 grams) has 92 Calories and 5 grams of fat. Certainly, the smaller snack bar is the better choice. Just be certain you know what you're going to do with the other 24 snack bars in that package, because those extra 2,200 Calories will be placed in your unwanted storage! Also, know how you are going to adjust the rest of your intake that day to account for the choice you are going to make. Once you read the label, you may decide that a walk around the lake, a walk in the zoo or Balboa Park and an iced cold glass of iced cold Sparkletts water, or Crystal Light lemonade would hit the stop just as nicely.

Be certain that what you have set as a goal will give you the satisfaction that you are seeking. Always keep your prime objective foremost in your mind's eye. Do you really want to lose 50 pounds, or do you really want to get away from your present, unhappy situation? Are you looking for that svelte healthy physique or simply more applause from the peanut gallery? Do you want to be thinner, or are you happy with the way things are now? Do you want better health, or are you simply looking for something to complain about? Is being overweight just one more reason to berate yourself for something that you thought that you should have achieved by now? Avoid self-pity! That is self destructive! Keep yourself riveted towards your target. Increase your effectiveness with intermediate goals. How, you say?

"I have too much to think about; the house, the kids my job, my husband, and my career." "What about my volunteer work at the hospital, my in-laws, and my parents? Let me point out something. If the rent or the mortgage is due, you pay it. It's either that or go into default or get evicted. If it's important, it gets done. No matter how many "more important" things are in your life now, getting yourself to a healthy weight once and for all ranks in the top three if not the top priority, because without your health, none of the rest matters! When you set an intermediate goal, you are merely reminding yourself to do something. You write yourself a note, when you've probably thought about doing some task for a period and it "didn't get done". When the mental note was ineffective, then you made an intermediate goal to get closer to accomplishing the goal you had set for yourself. Or you may give a goal so much importance, that you dare not forget it and you have used visualization without even thinking about how you did it. You painted a picture of the event in your mind with such clarity that you gave that intention a life of its own. You have made it a goal. Further, you have made a mental image of what you will do, and when you will do it. If you have a goal to accomplish and too many days go by with the task still undone, you will notice, your notes to yourself take a different form. For example, "Call the dentist for appointment, TODAY!"

Another example of intermediate goal setting is the planning that goes into taking a vacation. You are very careful to set intermediate goals to accomplish the final and primary goal. You won't find yourself writing a note. **"TAKE A VACATION"** You are anticipating time to relax. That's fun. What you have probably done, it circle the date on the calendar. You may have even sent for some brochures of the vacation place. You may find them in various places around the house. They may be tacked up on a board at work. You won't forget that! You're looking forward to it. In fact, for the last few days before your vacation, you may be mentally already there! You will have lists reminding you to get the tickets, arrange for the children's lessons, call to stop the paper, hold the mail. Do you see? You have been setting intermediate goals. It merely breaks down the larger goal into manageable steps. It assures that you will accomplish your primary goal.

So, write your intermediate goals. Substitute diet soda for regular soda, or buy Crystal Light. Buy bottled water to substitute for regular soda. Buy sugars substitutes or drink your coffee, or green tea without sweetener. The goal of weight reduction has more to do with substituting healthy habits for faulty ones, than it has to do about starving your self. When eating behaviors are controlled, then intake of high Calorie, fat laden snacks will be easier to control. But before you can change, you will need to know what habits need changing. Think about which foods you enjoy the most. When do you tend to snack? What time of the day, or what environment is most difficult to control.

"Out of sight, out of mind" works well. Take the cookies out of the cookie jar that scream COOKIES from across the room. Put them in the back of the cupboard. Buy air popped popcorn. A one-cup serving has 31 Calories and 1 gram of fiber.

Innovation is the key to reaching a goal that you want to achieve. Once you have set your goal, decide the best way to reach that goal, and then implement the plan. Teach yourself a positive a coping behavior. An innovative way to implement your plan is to decide the best way to get where you are going, through positive coping behaviors, and then put that plan into action. Change the behaviors that didn't work in the past, from destructive to productive. Whether its tobacco, alcohol, or overeating on a routine basis, these behaviors are additive and they are a method to cope with life's problems. To direct your behavior, alter the situation directly. Monitor the situation, and determine exactly what the stress in the situation is. It probably is not that the crying baby or your teenager who just asked to go who knows where. Look deeper. Was it the overdue bill in the mail? Did it confirm that you wouldn't be able to take that vacation after all? Was it your husband's phone call sharing his frustration over his current work situation, or a missed opportunity for the promotion? It usually is not the obvious irritant. It may take some searching. Then use your assertiveness to become more effective in dealing with the problem situation.

Use relaxation techniques to allow a stress free time to relax. When you take time to think, you will learn some things about your present situation that may surprise you. You will begin to realize the importance that you must place on all phases of your life. I had the very wonderful experience of spending four years in Japan. Japan, as you well know is a very small country, but out of that small country has come some extraordinary accomplishments. The Japanese people are able to compartmentalize their world. Focus on what you are doing when you are doing it to make your goals happen for you. Don't allow weight reduction to take a back seat. When you are focusing on portion control, or replacements for lower Calorie foods, make those activities top priority.

If negative thoughts keep you from acting, try the "picture, erase replace" technique of controlling your thoughts. See yourself at the buffet, but with too many high Calorie high fat choices. Take a deep breath of fresh air, and as you inhale, close your eyes and then exhale. As you exhale, erase the picture of failure. Now take in another deep breath. As you do, picture the changes in the scene, where you were tempted. Now see yourself substituting the nonfat frozen yogurt, or a fresh ripe peach. Watch as you replace the fat and Calorie ridden cheesecake back on the buffet table. See yourself as you place the salad dressing on the side and choose the grilled Sea Bass on a Ragout of Green lentils, spinach and wild mushroom truffles English pea puree, instead of fried fish tacos with a side order of super sized French fries.

Another worthwhile technique is to sit in a comfortable room and choose the most comfortable chair in the room. Picture yourself in a situation that is not necessarily pleasant. Close your eyes and envision the details of the unpleasant scene. Feel the feelings that come with the picture in this situation. Feel the discomfort. Now take the picture and move it farther away. See yourself step out of the picture, and move it just as if you were looking through a camera as you move the lens back, back away from where you are. Now make the picture smaller and smaller. See it as a picture on a postage stamp. Move it even farther away from you. Now make the picture darker. Make it black. Make the pinpoint of black smaller and smaller until it is smaller than the tip of a pen, a pinpoint, now smaller than a pinpoint…until it disappears. You have effectively erased the picture in your mind that is one of your stumbling blocks. Now bring back the picture. Are the feelings less intense? Repeat the steps again, until you feel a definite decrease in the intensity of the emotional impact on you. Continue to use these techniques to train yourself to decrease many of the daily stresses. You will find you have also addressed the irritants and have exercised more control in your world.

Now picture something that you perceive as pleasant and restful. It could be a picnic or any event where you are very much at ease. Notice your body position and your feelings. Now picture the event that gave you discomfort, dark and far away. Substitute the pleasant scene. Repeat this exercise until you feel more relaxed and in control. Use relaxation techniques to allow a stress free time to relax.

Remember to keep that positive self-image and the belief in the power that you hold the key to permanent weight loss, and control. You can use the relaxation sessions as a booster for reinforcement. Surround yourself with comfortable things such as comfortable lighting, music, and a cozy chair. When you are feeling down, take a bubble bath or a short nap to revitalize your energy. Do something that will take your mind off the stressful situation for a while. Go for a walk, or seek the company of a good friend, or a family member who has a listening ear and sympathetic understanding, and empathy. Read a book. If you feel the need, use your clergy or a mental health professional. Many times the problem can be worked out just by talking aloud to someone who cares to listen. Physical breaks may include going away for a vacation, or even for a week-end. Sometimes the change of scenery or by moving from one place to another will help you put the problem into perspective. Take a ride in the car or on a bus or walk in the park or out in the country, or the desert. To give yourself the greatest chance for personal success, take the time to analyze your personal situation. Although you may not be able to change all the things that are causing stress, it may surprise you that even changing one or two things will make the problems that seemed insurmountable, less important. Don't let weight management take a back seat. Give this project your undivided attention; Follow the keys until you feel more power over any self-destructive moods. That is specifically those little devils that tell you can't do it. Use stimulus control to manage your eating activities and master your eating patterns. You must continue to believe that the changes you are making are beneficial. Learn to understand the eating patterns that will help you attain your goal.

As the New Year rings in, millions of Americans will make a New Year's resolution to make a positive weight change, to improve their health. It is important to make sure those goals are reasonable. They should be goals that can be met, and kept through healthy changes in eating. Simple changes are the most effective. The loftier the goal, the easier it is to break. Use the intermediate goals to accomplish your primary purpose and goal. Think of ways to increase the intake of fresh fruit, and vegetables daily. Change from regular to diet soda. Begin to make time for a walk daily. Buy 1% low fat milk instead of 2% milk. Or buy 2% low fat milk instead of whole milk. Start the day right with breakfast. A simple bowl of cereal will qualify. Fresh fruit and yogurt is another good choice. Remember breakfast will help you avoid the tempting high fat doughnuts at work.

Finally, develop your own support system. People in your world have a powerful effect upon your actions. This can work in both a positive and negative sense. It has been said that seeds of destruction are planted unknowingly by well meaning but ignorant comments of significant others. But a significant other is not necessarily a mother, father, sister, brother. It could very well be a bus driver, a janitor, a school teacher a clerk in a store. It's amazing how much influence the words of adults have on children in our world.

Surround yourself with the positive players. While the dynamics of relationships are beyond the scope of this book, the perceived support or sabotage from significant others can be the difference between success and failure. Learn to develop an effective and positive support system. Want to win! A winner needs a goal, a plan and a strategy. Want to develop that smaller waistline, that lower pulse rate that increases in fitness and higher energy level, and improved health. Set a specific goal in terms of pounds that you want to lose. Take a pen and paper and write that down. Then, go one step further. Set intermediate goals in terms of timeline to attain your primary goal. Know what your plan is to reach your goal.

Use the support of your significant others to begin to follow a healthy lifestyle change. Use problem solving to find ways to handle difficult times and avoid unnecessary stumbling blocks. Don't do too much too soon. Many of your responses to food are learned responses. Remember Pavlov and the learned response. The dog did not salivate the first time Pavlov rang the bell. He "learned" to salivate only when he found the bell was associated with dinner. When you see a commercial for Burger King, do you begin to get hungry for a fast food snack? Advertising brings food to our attention. New products virtually unknown on the market can become an overnight success with advertising. Food companies influence our choices in countless blunt and subtle ways. How many times have you driven by a fast food restaurant and been enticed by the aroma of the burgers? Don't think of it as a wonderful reminder that you might need a snack. Redefine it as a diabolical scheme by big business to pry your money from your purse, and clog your arteries with trans fat. It might not hurt your bottom line, but it will definitely affect your bottom.

It's difficult to measure the influence of the advertisements in our food choices but it is inexplicably intertwined with our lifestyle.

"The burgers are better..."

"...helps build strong bodies..."

"...have it your way..."

Food advertising encourages overeating. It directs weight conscious consumers to purchase special "diet" foods, or foods that are "low fat", "carbohydrate controlled" or "Lite".

These foods are more expensive and usually unnecessary. Colorful and beautifully photographed food advertisements create a desire to eat that food for breakfast, lunch and dinner. The food companies have attained their objective…to sell their food to you. They really don't care if you don't need the extra calories as long as they get their market share of your dollar. You've been taught just like Pavlov's dog, by the advertising. You too have developed a learned response to the dinner bell. Begin to "unlearn" those sounds and smells that tell you there is "dinner" at the end of the maze. When you "unlearn" those negative influences, you will begin to feel the power in your world and you will be on your way to a slimmer and healthier you. Smile! If you think you can, you can!

Feel the power in your world and see the path to success using your positive cognitive ecology. Reject the idea that food is a comfort. Food does not make holidays special. People make holidays special. Food is not a comfort. Don't let it be your crutch!

Nutrition Knowledge Check

Check your current level of nutrition knowledge with this short quiz.

1. Most weight problems are inherited.
2. A person hose parents are overweight or who has been overweight since childhood is probably naturally overweight.
3. Hormone problems, particularly thyroid deficiencies are responsible for many cases of obesity.
4. You should expect to gain more weight as you get older. It's natural.
5. "I'm just big boned.

ANSWERS:

1, 2, 3. You can't always blame it on your ancestors. Since the tendency for weight problems seems to run in families, it may be that you inherit a predisposition to become heavy. But the real answer is that is it difficult to separate the influence of genes from the environment. "Fat families" share the same genetic heritage, as well as the same food habits. So the more important question is, did you inherit your mother's weight problem, or rather did you learn to be passive about activity, indulge in too many high calorie snacks, eat at fast food restaurants too often, and eat too much of your mother's "good" cooking? Scientists who have researched the question of nature versus nurture using twins who were adopted by different families and by comparing foster children's weights with their natural parents suggest that your genes load the gun and the environmental influences pull the trigger. So if you come from a long line of overweight people, don't despair. Instead realize you can control you future by developing healthy eating and activity habits. You can still become thin in a "fat" family.

4. it's true that most Americans gain 15 to 25 pounds after the age of 25, even when their eating habits don't change. The most likely explanation for this is that over time people become less active. As family age there is less running around for family and job related activities. There is less planned exercise such as tennis, or golf. Younger family members do the chores like mowing the lawn, which results in fewer calories used. Additionally, there is some evidence that for each decade after the age of forty, your basal energy expenditure (the energy that you need to keep your heart, lungs, brain, kidneys, and liver all working decreases by about 10%.

5. To determine if your frame is small, medium or large. Take your dominant hand try to touch your index finger and thumb by wrapping your hand around the wrist of your non-dominant hand. Be sure to encircle your wrist just below the ulna bone. If your thumb and your index finger overlap, you are small framed. If your thumb and your index finger just meet, you are medium framed and if your thumb and your index finger don't touch, then you are large framed. This is not the most accurate and to increase accuracy you should use a tape measure but it will give you a gross estimator. Knowing your actual frame size might surprise you!

Chapter 3

What You Eat You Are
Carbohydrates, Fat and Protein;
Time in the Counting House

What is a Calorie? A Calorie is the unit of heat measured to burn a food completely to ash in a bomb calorimeter. Foods are made of at least one and possibly as many as three fuel nutrients. These food constituents are burned by the body to release energy to keep our body going. These three fuel nutrients are carbohydrate, fat and protein. When any of these fuel nutrients are burned the energy that is released in units of heat called Calories fuels our body to do the days work. Carbohydrates are the body's preferred source of energy. Protein is used for growth, repair and maintenance. Both carbohydrate and protein provide 4 calories of energy per gram of food used. The amount of energy provided by fat is over twice as high as carbohydrate or protein. It provides nine Calories per gram of fat burned.

To lose one pound in one week, you will need to avoid 3500 Calories, or an average of 500 Calories a day. That is two 12 oz. sodas, and a small bag of potato chips. That's not much, you say. Yet, in year, like putting money in the bank, the reverse is also true, and you have accumulated 52 pounds (182,000 Calories) of ugly fat. You can eat five hundred less Calories than you need, and in seven short days, you can reverse the storage procedure, and lose one pound of fat. You need only know how much you need, and this procedure will work for you.

Where can I find 500 calories to avoid? Where do the Calories come from?

"That's easy." You say. They come from baked, stuffed lobster, and shrimp. They come from Bavarian Waffles, and Danish pastries, and ice cream, cake and pies. But what is it in those foods that makes them high calorie? How can you easily identify the problem foods and avoid them. Or once identified, eat them in such small amounts that the discretionary Calories will not sabotage your weight loss plans?

When you eat a product with both carbohydrates and fat where the carbohydrate has been concentrated by cooking, the number of total Calories can be significantly higher than without cooking. That is where label reading becomes an essential tool. Nutrient density is an indication of how many nutrients that you get in a food product per Calorie. Just check any product to see the quality that you get for your dollar. The nutrient value you get from a food should be equally important to you. Donuts can be as low as 125 Calories for a plain, cakelike donut, or over 225 Calories for a raised or yeast donut with a jelly filling. It can be higher for a chocolate cream filled donut. A slice of whole wheat bread can be as low as 65 Calories per slice, or it can be as high as 80 Calories for a slice of potato bread. Think about what you are getting as you reach for the convenience of high Calorie, high fat, and concentrated carbohydrate foods.

Budget your Calories, just as you budget your money. Finally, you must realize that all the diets in the world will not work for you unless you control your mental attitude towards food. The only way to succeed is to get your positive cognitive ecology in gear. Reject the attitude that food is a comfort. Food doesn't make holidays special! Food is not a comfort, and don't let it be your crutch!

Obesity is an obsolete term. It was meant to be a greater weight than normal. But what is "normal". Total weight includes muscle, bone, and fat. If, then, a person is athletic, he or she may have a higher muscle composition, and hence be "overweight". Truly, the individual is not over "fat" for his or her particular body type and the distribution of types of tissue within the body. The total amount of his or her particular body type and the type of tissue may actually be lower than the assumed "normal". Are you at an ideal weight for your height according to the Metropolitan Life or Body Mass Index tables? What exactly is ideal body weight anyway?

If you are over 200% of ideal body weight you are considered morbidly obese. If you are considered over 130% over ideal weight you are obese. If you are 110-120% over ideal boy weight you are considered overweight.

I can't tell you how many people, when I suggest what the Metropolitan Life standard, or the BMI standard is their "normal or ideal weight" have said,

"I've never weighed that!" Or maybe they have said,

"I think I might have weighed that, but I was sick."

Obesity, that ugly word, has come to replace overweight and specifies the type of weight as an accumulation of body fat or adipose tissue, with an excessive proportion to total body mass. People have advanced arguments for the tendency towards fatness and offer the morphology of cows; the Angus versus the Jersey. Both cows are certainly entirely different body types. Granted, but let's take a closer look and analyze what the farmer does to enhance these two body types. Environmental factors are part of this equation. There is lifestyle, diet, stress and the race to the kitchen between television commercials to be considered.

Obesity has been defined as 15-20% above the "normal" weight with 10% of the weight from fat or adipose tissue. It has also been defined as 130% of "normal or ideal" body weight. Obesity arises from interrelationships of psychological, physiological, environmental, and genetic factors. Today 55% of adult Americans are overweight or obese. Statistics tell us that the number of deaths related to obesity climbs yearly. In this world of societal evils; canapé's, cocktails, sumptuous gourmet meal, fast foods, and the endless snack foods available obesity is taking its toll. It is evidenced in hypertension, diabetes, and heart disease. In fact, statistics tell us that this generation may be the first not to outlive their parents. That number one killer is intimately linked to obesity. It's no secret; we Americans are eating ourselves into an early grave. But what are we to do about it? To find out what you shouldn't eat, just pick up any magazine, or newspaper. Google the question and you will come up with hundreds of answers.

"Don't eat salt."

"Avoid too much fat, especially the trans fats and saturated fats."

"Avoid eggs."

"Avoid dairy products because they are high in saturated fats."

"Dairy products have been shown in recent studies to actually help with weight loss, (probably paid for by the Dairy Council.)

"Eggs are okay." (Probably paid for by the Egg Council)

"Give up caffeine."

"Caffeine, in moderation is okay. (probably paid for by the Caffeine Council.)

"Give up chocolate."

"Chocolate has been shown in recent research to be good for you." (probably paid for by the Chocolate Council.)

To identify the foods that are the freshest and are the highest nutrient density, buy the foods that are advertised the least. When was the last time that you saw an advertisement for brussel sprouts, spinach, or broccoli, eggplant, cabbage or green beans? Yet, these fresh vegetables are high in essential minerals, and the water soluble vitamin B complex vitamins. These are vitamins that are needed in our diets daily because there is no body storage of these nutrients. Too, these vegetables are highest in total fiber. Grandma called it roughage and it becomes lower in our diets as we substitute the more highly processed and more highly advertised foods that are available through the miracles of modern technology.

Should we give up every delicacy? Every sweet morsel of food? Alternatively, we could go to the health food store and pay outrageous prices for "organic" foods with some assurance of wholesomeness or quality. But would that guarantee that we will become somehow thin? Nonsense! What we must do is learn to eat sensibly, today. Excess fats or excess sugars in our diet tend to add extra calories and unwanted pounds. Simple sugars elevate triglycerides (blood fat) and are now being implicated in several cancers. To painlessly eliminate extra fat from your diet, watch out for the sneaky calories that are in salad dressings, sauces, gravies, fried foods, and rich high fat, high sugar desserts.

But before you change anything, STOP. Avoid the "Swallow it Whole Theory". Don't change anything until you are ready. Just as there is no average American, there is no ideal diet for anyone. Sit down in a quiet corner and assess you lifestyle and how you feel. Look at the things that need changing and work at changing one habit at a time. That means you must learn about the food you eat.

The first key to sensible eating is know exactly what you are eating in terms of Calories, carbohydrate, protein and fat in a particular portion of that food. When you have accomplished that, you can eat anything you want. Notice the word is anything, not "as much as'" then, if you have decided to have two portions of that particular something, know what the caloric and nutrient consequences are. Once you have discovered the truth, you may be only to glad to "just have one". If you usually order an extra large, you may be tempted to order a small. You are the person in control. You are the customer, and the customer is always right!

What is a calorie? Put quite simply, a calorie is a measurement of heat. To find the number of calories in a particular food, the food is placed in a bomb calorimeter and burned to ash. The amount of heat is recorded and the amount of heat required to burn the food completely is measured in kilocalories. One thousand calories is equal to one Calorie (or one kilocalorie).

What then are the fuel nutrients? There are three categories of fuel nutrients; carbohydrates, fat and protein. These fuel nutrients when burned give off energy. Carbohydrates, and proteins yield four calories per gram of food burned, and fat yields nine calories per gram of food burned. If you drink ethanol then these calories yield seven calories per gram and are metabolized similarly to fats.

Where do we find carbohydrates, fats, and protein in the foods we eat?

Carbohydrates are the preferred source of energy and are found in breads, grains, and cereals, fruits and fruit juices, starchy vegetables such as peas, lima beans, and lentils, corn, potatoes, winter squash, rice and yams and dairy products such as milk, soy milk, and yogurt.

Very simply, your weight state is controlled by eating and the balance or imbalance between what you eat and what energy you use in a day. Energy intake can increase because of an increase in total food intake or by increasing the calorie density of the foods that we eat. When patients tell me,

"I really don't eat that much."

That's no surprise! You don't have to eat that much, to eat too many calorie dense foods without realizing it. For instance, you've decided to have a snack of popcorn you want to munch on five cups. Now keep in mind that is five 8 ounce measuring cups, not overflowing, but even at the 8 ounce level.

Air popped white popcorn has 155 Calories, 11 grams of fiber, 1.7 grams of fat.

Cheese flavored popcorn has 290 Calories, 5.5 grams of fiber, 18.25 grams of fat.

Carmel coated popcorn has 847 Calories, 8 grams of fiber, 16.5 grams of fat.

You can see that the more processed the food is, the more Calories are contributed from fat, and simple sugars. Additional sugars will contribute extra calories. You can also see that as the food is more processed the amount of fiber in the product decreases. Remember, to keep the integrity of that concept, you cannot add melted butter (saturated fat calories) to the air popped popcorn without adding Calories but you can add garlic powder or onion powder to enhance the taste without the Calories.

We have too much food to choose from. We produce millions of tons of products in this breadbasket of the world. Unfortunately, nutrition education in our schools is not one of the three R's. So health conscious Americans listen to any and all advice on how to make molehills out of their mountains, no matter how incomplete, or totally erroneous. There are over 30, 00 methods of weight loss and control that contribute to the multi-billion dollar diet industry. Sadly, however, over half of these methods are backed by nutrition fraud, misinformation, and fad diets. We need a weight control bible that works. Simple nutrition principles accurately applied can spell the difference between obesity and healthy, effective weight management.

In grammar school, we learned our alphabet, we learned to add, subtract, multiply and divide. We learned how to write our names, and to make grammatically correct sentences. But somehow, when we were preparing our youth to care for themselves, we forgot to tell our children that there are three fuel nutrients; carbohydrate, fat and protein. (This is discounting alcohol which will be discussed later) In the energy equation carbohydrates and protein contribute four Calories in each gram and fat contributed over twice as much with 9 Calories in each gram. We didn't tell our youth that carbohydrates are the preferred source of energy for the body and that the natural fiber, both soluble and insoluble will help to even out our glucose curve, decrease the serum cholesterol levels in our body, act as if having anti-cancer properties, provide important nutrients, and bulk for peristalsis. We neglected to mention how important it is to include fiber in our diets by snacking on fresh fruits and vegetables, and using water when we are thirsty instead of sweet, high calorie sodas.

We didn't impress upon our youth that protein is important for growth, repair and maintenance of our tissues, but since that is its function, we don't want to overburden our systems with more protein than we need for metabolism. We never mentioned that Calories in must equal Calories out or we will gain weight. We let food manufacturers do that teaching. And teach us they did. The food industry coupled incomplete knowledge of food facts and nutrition with powerful advertising dollars in the food industry. By the 1980s, the advertising message was clear. Fast food became a way of life and the sum is a nation where 60% of the population is overweight and 31% of the people are frankly obese.

Very simply then, eating is controlled by balance or imbalance between what you eat and the energy you use in a day. But the problems of overeating are complex.

"It looks too good to resist." That is your favorite company at work to make their advertising pay off in their fiercely competitive market, to make you spend your money for their product, to sell you a piece of their pie.

Eating is a habit, a learned behavior, taught by advertising dollars. Overweight and obesity are the consequences and are attached to the stigma of a judgmental society obsessed with thinness. Obesity is commonly assessed to be the result of laziness and a lack of self control. The psychological burden that attitude imposes can have far reaching consequences on overall mental health and well being. The driving urge should be to become healthy. Think about the reasons you want to lose weight now. Is it because you feel uncomfortable? It has to be more than that! Is there medical pressure to reduce? Whatever the reason, the final and most important reason must come from inside. Think back to the last diet. Something motivated you to pick up the diet book, or put down the fork. Something motivated you to begin to watch what you are eating, and to begin to read the labels on foods you bought. Do you want to fit into that new bikini? Do you want to fit into that prom dress, that wedding dress? Do you want to be alive and healthy enough to be able to crawl on the floor with your grandchildren?

Since you've established that you want to lose weight, the first step towards success is to know thyself and the food you eat. Life patterns like eating patterns are learned, and any faulty habits must be unlearned. But, before you begin those changes you must find out exactly what needs changing. Success comes in many forms. No matter what shape or size you're in you can be successful. Success means achieving the right weight and eating pattern to maintain that weight. It means taking an honest look at yourself and map out the steps to improve your patterns for long term success. That success is built one day at a time, like a small savings account, it means putting good habits and good feelings about you in your computer brain. It means feeling good about you from the inside out.

You must know exactly where you eat, and with whom you munch those morsels that you are consuming. Once you are aware of the habits that you have acquired, divide those habits into habits that need changing, and those worth keeping. When you know what motivates you may be surprised to find that its the time of day, the atmosphere, the sound of music, the alarm clock, boredom, depression, even restlessness. External cues often signal "time to eat" but are not signals of true physiological hunger.

Once you have identified external cues, you can more easily substitute the healthy habits for the faulty ones, or alter the environment to eliminate the motivators. We don't just sit down to eat. Something motivates us. Reasons we eat are associated with the sight, smell, touch, and thoughts of food. Further, the only person who can record this accurately is you. You may not have a degree in Nutrition, but you have been living with habits that you developed for your entire lifetime. Today is the time to stop and look at those habits.

We all expect miracles. We all want to win the lotto. We hear about miracles in church. We see miracles on television, and in the movies. We expect no less in our weight management efforts. To tell the world that there is no miracle solution and no short cut to weight control is to destroy the American dream. If you were admitted to a hospital, and placed on a strict weight reduction program, you would lose weight temporarily. But in the final analysis, it is you, who to maintain that weight loss, must exert self knowledge and management in your every day world. Presently, I will ask you to keep several records of your daily activities. These are for you. Now, make a promise to be totally honest with yourself in your record keeping. I will not ask you to decrease the amount you are eating in one day, just to record it accurately. Let's check your present weight state.

What was your lowest adult weight?   What year was that?

What was your highest adult weight?   What year was that?

If you consider yourself overweight now, when did you begin to realize that you were over your ideal weight range?

Did your weight fluctuate when you were married or divorced?

If you were pregnant, did you lose the extra weight after your pregnancy ended?

Any life changes are times when there if a possibility of weight fluctuations. It may be an indication of changing stress situations, or changes in activity, the key here is change. Whenever your routine is disrupted, the results may be a weight change. Use a chart to check if you are close to an acceptable weight range for your height. For example, if you a woman who is 5'4" without your shoes, you will find that your average weight is 120 pounds.

Further, there is a range from 108 to 138. To see, where in that range you would be most comfortable check your frame. Too many times people have said, "But I have a large frame..." You can check this too. A somewhat inaccurate, but easy method is the following. Simply measure the size of your wrist, at its smallest circumference, just in front of your ulna bone at the beginning of your wrist. Then compare the frame size for your height without shoes. If, according to the chart your wrist measures less than 6" you are indeed a small frame, and your weight range would be 108-118#. If your frame was medium; that is your wrist measured between 6-6 1/4", then your ideal weight range would be 118-128 pounds. Similarly, if your wrist measured 6 1/4" or more then you would be most comfortable in the 118-128 pound range. Setting a goal weight is not about perfection, as much as progress. It isn't about being a size 4 or size 6. You may feel terrific as a size 10. Forget about the ideal and focus on improvements.

If you find your height and think that the weight seems unreasonably high or unreasonably low you may have other parameters that need to be considered.

For example, you may have a large portion of muscle mass. This does make a difference. If you're extremely muscular, or an athletic individual, your weight may vary well over what the table indicates you should weigh. That is because your muscle mass is larger than an individual who is not athletic. Lean tissue weighs more than fat or adipose tissue, and if you are athletic, it should not alarm you to weigh slightly more. You may notice that skinny kids seem to work very hard to keep afloat while swimming, while a large, overweight woman paddles serenely along without much effort to stay afloat. Fat floats. If you throw a cube of butter into a swimming pool, it will float just like an ice cube. Pour oil onto water. The body fat is no different. The more fat you have, the better you float. Remember, it is the amount of FAT tissue that you want to control. Muscle contours the body. Now, do some simple arithmetic:

My actual weight_____Date_____

My goal weight_____

Pounds to lose_____to reach my weight maintenance goal.

Subtract your actual weight from your goal weight to find how many pounds that you will want to lose permanently. I can hear the sighs from here! Don't become discouraged, that is just a number. Now that you have a specific number of pounds that you will ultimately lose, you're ready to begin.

How long did it take you to put on the excess weight? If you think about it, you probably gained it in the same way that you have built up your net worth in your savings account, by putting, small, unused deposits of calories into your adipose tissue account. You didn't wake up one morning fat! No matter what your pattern is, this will be beneficial to you in your weight reduction. Trickling down to your ideal weight is the realistic approach. The majority of us have seen an extra tire or two around the waist, felt an inch too many in the pinch, or maybe caught a glimpse of a forming double chin. Now, the state of things has been defined. Take responsibility.

You are in control, and you can do something about your own weight state, today. To become thin, you must know how, and which foods to be most cautious of. You must further be aware of the reasons why you are overweight now. Knowledge is power, and once you have the basic knowledge and know which foods to be the most cautious about, you will be in more complete control of your life situation. Your habits may be just routine actions that you never have thought too much about. If food habits are found to be associated with something that is emotionally or ethnically tied to your background, the change will require more effort, even when change is recommended for health reasons. Then, the primary goal in weight reduction and control is not the elimination of all the "favorite foods". This is not a mini course in self-deprivation. This is merely a readjustment of how you perceive these foods; how important these foods really are to your life and what exactly they stand for. It is the understanding, and choice for control. At last, it is a final, honest look at what these foods really stand for! Remember, weight loss is secondary; the control of your intake is primary. Once behavior is understood, you are better able to control the foods you eat. When the results are positive, your understanding makes intake control more positive. Healthy habits substituted for fat habits will continue to teach and reinforce control over an extended period of time. When you respond to stress, you may respond by eating. For change to happen in this pattern, it is first most important to know the pattern, in an attempt to understand and alter the stress situation or alter your response to the stress.

Success will come in small steps. As long as you involve yourself in practice as you become more knowledgeable about the foods you eat, and the reasons that you eat them. You WANT to lose weight, and first you will find the most success by controlling the portion sizes of the foods that you eat. Remember the switch from cola to diet drinks, or even water, the original diet drink! Work for short term change. Take an amount of time that is manageable for you. One day is not a lifetime. It the first small step towards your goal. Pinpoint a problem area.

Sally used to nibble on Fritos when she read the paper each evening. She consumed nearly a package every time she read the news! Do you know how many calories that represented? In a six ounce package there are over five hundred Calories. If it takes three thousand five hundred calories to make one pound of fat, then in just 7 days of eating one six ounce package, she could accumulate enough Calories to make one pound of ugly, body fat! But, you say,

"I understand she needed something to munch on..." Why not try sugarless gum.

It may not look demure, but neither does an individual who could be a size twelve, instead of the sloppy size twenty. What price "something to munch on"?

Mrs. M., a widow, while in counseling reported that she considered the high point of her day, mail time. She would wait for the mail, while nibbling, take a snack when she walked down the drive to get the mail, and then while she opened the mail, she would munch on cookies, cake or "whatever was around". She had programmed her eating responses to the event of the mail. Over a period of months she had become very much overweight. She needed to shift gears and reprogram her response. She substituted rice cakes which she didn't particularly crave, while she was working through the reasons for the habits that she had developed. The calories that she saved were enough to allow Mrs. M. to lose forty-five pounds in a matter of only six months.

What she discovered when she went through the analysis, she was alone, and for the first time in years she realized that the food was replacing the companionship and love of her husband she had recently lost. Thankfully, once she had realized that, she was able to redirect herself to seek friendship in Bingo, a dance group and other social activities, so that those friends and not the mail became the focus of her life.

The next step is work. What small steps can you take today to reduce or substitute a food? You never heard about all the work that it took that little train who thought he could, to pull that big engine over the hill. You only heard about what he had his mind set to do. He thought he could! Don't kid yourself. That was work! But the train thought, and you think that it's worth the effort to succeed. What does it take to control your actions? Understand what you do, why you do it, why it's important and then think what could you substitute? Begin to break the old, faulty behavior, by developing a new, more beneficial habit. Before you make any significant change, ask first,

"Can I handle this, just for today? Do you want to do it? Believe it and you can do it. You will help yourself by becoming aware of what your eating patterns routinely are.

Identify your favorite foods and your usual eating patterns. Who cooks most of the meals? This is important. The individual who cooks the meals has the most control over the total caloric contribution that they provide to the eater. How many people the meals are prepared for? Have the total number of people varied. If this is true the chef may be preparing the same number of meals as if there were several other family members.

A nurse came to me with a good deal of concern about her significant weight gain. She said that she had taken Nutrition classes in nursing school, she knew about Nutrition, and she didn't see how it would help to talk to me. However, since her endocrinologist insisted, she made an appointment. After some questioning, she said that she had two sons; one had just joined the Navy, and a second was in his first year at college. When I asked how many people that she prepared meals for it became apparent that although she and her husband were the only two left at home, she was still preparing meals for four! The only problem was that since she didn't like to save leftovers, she and her husband were eating the entire amount that had been prepared. Needless to say, once the portion sizes were reduced, both she and her husband were able to lose weight easily.

Make it your business to know portion sizes and control them. Particularly become familiar with the common household measures of the teaspoon, and the tablespoon. Find how much is in a handful, especially YOUR handful. Get a postal scale, or small scale that will measure ounces. The next time you are preparing dinner, measure one ounce of beef. Examine that amount. Not much is it? Next measure three ounces and make it into a patty. Take a piece of lunch meat, and weigh that to be sure that it isn't more than one ounce. Take a chicken leg and weigh it with the bone. Now remove the bone and weigh the poultry only. Look in your freezer, and check the fish and chicken you have purchased. What is the total purchased in ounces and pounds of the package? How many are you expecting that to serve? If you are allowing more than three or four ounces per serving, rethink your serving sizes.

Finally compare the size of the portion to the sizes served in the restaurants. What a difference! A popular restaurant in town that specializes in steak advertises a 16 ounce sirloin steak. That one serving of steak provides the RDI (Recommended Daily Intake) for protein of a 246 pound individual for one day! Now, that you are aware, it will make more sense to split a meal with a friend, or ask for that "doggie bag" to allow yourself a sane meal out, as well as enjoying a second meal "out" at home.

Are you ready to set a goal? Set one that is easy, and you cannot fail to do. It can be as simple as a substitution. Don't start tomorrow. Tomorrow never comes. Decide to do it for a finite period of time, not for a week or a month or a year. Simply to do it for one day…today.

When filling out the information on your average intake, and frequency, the key is regularly. It's not the broiled live lobster that will hurt; it's the drawn butter that you dip the lobster in before you savor it. It's the margarine or the butter or sour cream that you use routinely on potatoes. It's the butter that melts into the rolls in the restaurant. It's not the Christmas eggnog, unless it's more than once each year. It's the whipped cream on the Jell-O, and the cream or nondairy coffee creamer in those four cups of coffee that you have each morning. To get an accurate picture of those foods that are high in fat, that you use every day, write a food diary and record, record, record!

Make it your business to learn about portion sizes. I can't tell you how many people I have counselled who are certain the portion sizes of their foods are exactly ½ cup portions, or that their glass of juice in the morning is "about 4 ounces." What is the most helpful is visualization. I have a set of measuring cups in my office. You have seen these in any supermarket. There is a ¼ cup, 1/3 cup, ½ cup and 1 cup measure. When an individual is asked how much orange juice he or she has in the morning the answer is inevitably,

"A little glass…" But when I ask them to estimate according to the measuring cups, how much they drink, it is often 8-10 ounces and frequently as much as 12 ounces. To make matters more confusing, when the USDA developed label standards, sadly, they chose no standardization for portion sizes. So manufacturers, eager to sell and re-sell their product determined what a serving size of their product is and for many juices it is 8 ounces. This is contrary to the American Diabetes Association determination of serving size which they say is 4 ounces.

In one serving determined by the manufacturer to be 8 ounces of orange juice, fresh, California chilled, there are 110 Calories, and 25 grams of carbohydrate and no dietary fiber. But in one piece of fresh fruit, a raw California Valencia about 2 5/8 inches in diameter, there are 59 Calories, 3 grams of dietary fiber, and 14 grams of carbohydrate. It's to the manufacturer's advantage to determine the serving size to be twice what one fruit juiced would provide. That way they will ultimately sell the product they brought to the marketplace twice as fast, because they have set a serving size that is advantageous to them and will sell their product twice as fast. Make it your business to know what the portion size is for every product you consume. And while you are looking, see how many Calories that represents. Use an ordinary household measure. Once you know what and how much you are eating, it's easier to decide to have a smaller serving or to allow yourself to have the larger amount without feeling guilty about it.

The next thing that you should do is take your ordinary household measuring cup and fill it with one cup (8 ounces) of tap water. Now pour that amount of water into your favorite drinking cup or glass. Is it more or less than four ounces? Do the same with your juice glass. The measurement becomes particularly critical when you are filling your cup with a fluid that is high in sodium or a salty food such tomato or vegetable juice. Although sodium has no Calories, it causes the body to retain fluid. Then, when you lose fat weight, the body with larger sodium intakes will tend to retain fluid, and the scale won't record that positive weight loss as readily. That is never advantageous. It tends to mark a failure on the part of the dieter or the diet book and the end to "that diet". Higher sodium intakes will also decrease the effectiveness of your high blood pressure medications.

Regularly give yourself the praise you deserve in any number of changes you are making in the types of foods that you eat daily. Did you know that merely switching from regular twelve ounce cola or soda to water can save over 150 Calories?

If you are ingesting an excessive amount of caffeine and decide to give it up you may actually suffer withdrawal symptoms unless you decrease the amount gradually over a period of time. How much is too much? An eight ounce cup of brewed coffee contains from 10-40 milligrams of caffeine, depending on the strength, and the type of coffee. Dripolated coffee usually weaker, and the freeze-dried or instant varieties vary from 55-65 milligrams per cup. A cardiovascular and sports nutritionist in the Boston area, author of "The Athlete's Kitchen" considers over 250 milligrams daily excessive. How much caffeine have you had today? You might be surprised, not only does coffee, and cola drinks contain caffeine, but it's also found in chocolate, soft candy, and puddings. Don't forget that some over the counter medications for headache, and cold remedies contain caffeine as well.

Alcohol contributes additional calories and if the cocktail, or beer is more than an occasional occurrence, the calories can become the stumbling block to any good weight reduction program.

Chapter 4

PREPLANNING TO AVOID THE STUMBLING BLOCKS

Weigh yourself on your scale. You say you don't know how much you weigh, and you don't have a scale? The first order of business is to buy one. Don't get fancy. Any ordinary bathroom scale will do. To eliminate deviations, however, you will be weighing yourself on the same scale, at the same time of day. The preferred time to weigh is before breakfast, in the morning a la birthday suit. The majority of us have seen an extra tire, or left an extra inch in the pinch around your waist and maybe caught the glimpse of the forming double chin. Now that we have defined the state of things generally, make the decision. Decide you are worth the effort to work towards a better healthy state. You are going to begin to reduce the excess baggage and shape up what's left. Learn your desirable weight for your height. Notice that your height measurements are without shoes. Now write down your healthy weight range from the lowest to the highest. For example, if you are a woman who is five feet and five inches tall, your ideal range will be 111-142 pounds.

Take a look at your plan, and the influences that control your life. Obesity is a matter of balance. Many people have a balancing plan, a plan that hasn't worked in the past. Many factors can influence your plan, and modify your normal energy balance. It may be environmental, heredity, emotional or the result of your coping mechanisms that you have derived for yourself over the years. There may be an elevated level of beta endorphin which inducing overeating. Additionally, endogenous opiates regulate the pain sensation, and may actually induce eating. The pain threshold in overweight and obese individuals appears to be higher than in normal weight individuals. The television shows have changed over the years, but the television ads haven't. You can still see fit, trim models eating high calorie, high fat foods and snacks, but miraculously maintain their svelte figures. This mistakenly fuels the misconception that its possible to eat like the typical American yet still maintain the body of the American idol. Most weight reducers enormously underestimate the number of Calories that we eat in a day. Just a quick snack at McDonald's of a Big Mac with Cheese, 5 ½ ounce serving of fries, and a 13 ½ ounce Chocolate Shake will cost you 1620 Calories. This may be more Calories than you burn in an entire day. More, we tend to over estimate the number of Calories that we burn up. One of the patients that I saw was very conscious of the things that she ate and recounted what she ate with extreme accuracy.

"At lunchtime", she said, "I always eat in the hospital cafeteria, and I have the salad bar."

"What do you put on the salad?" I asked.

"The Thousand Islands dressing", she added.

"How much?"

"Just two of those little ladles."

This patient had just unknowingly identified the fact that she put over 400 Calories onto her salad everyday, or enough to add one extra pound of body weight to her frame every nine days, which, by the way was about what she was gaining. You see, she didn't realize the number of Calories that can be packed into any fat. Karen laughed and commented,

"So much for my weight reduction plan..." That's very healthy! Always remember to laugh at yourself. If you can't laugh at your failings, learn by your mistakes. Massage your self esteem and start anew. What you consider a weakness is merely ignorance, or an overextension of what you are expecting of yourself. You have a career, in which you probably excel. You are probably not a registered dietitian. You didn't fail. You succeeded in finding one more way to avoid gaining weight that you don't want. With what you know, make the commitment to change. Use vinegar, rice wine vinegar, or lemon wedges to moisten your salad, or a scoop of cottage cheese on top of your salad. Then, use the dressing of your choice on the side in a small cup. Dip your fork into the dressing and then into the salad. You may be surprised how much less dressing you will use and more, what that unnecessary salad dressing was contributing in terms of unwanted calories. Respond with productivity not depression, and look again at your plan. Plan ahead before you begin eating. Rediscover what you usually eat and drink. How much? How long does it take you? Who is with you? Then use the stimulus control method to manage your eating activities, and master your eating habits. Think of the response to the smell of food, and to the taste. Do you eat routinely after seven PM.? For one week hang a "NO EATING AFTER 7PM" sign in the kitchen. Are you a snacker? What is your favorite? Sweets or salty snacks? Hang a "NO SNACKS" sign up. Then, think again, about Pavlov and his experiment. Remember the dog did not salivate at the first bell ring. He "learned" to salivate only when he found that the bell was the dinner bell. Begin to "unlearn" those negative cues, those sounds that tell you there is food at the en of the maze. When you "unlearn" those negative responses, you will begin to feel power in your world and you will be on your way to a slimmer you. That should make you smile. If you think you can...YOU CAN!

"How many appetizers or drinks will I have?"
"What would really taste good?"
"If I don't want to avoid a high Calorie food, can you only eat part of it?"
"Can I save a portion in a "doggie bag"?

For breakfast, if you decide to have two poached eggs, three strips of bacon, eight ounces of whole, homogenized milk, you would be starting out with breakfast amounting to 78+78+46+46+46+160 = 448 Calories. But if instead you had ONE poached egg, one strip of bacon, and eight ounces of fat free or skim milk, the figures would be altered. The result would be 201 Calories. Notice you didn't change what you ate. We only changed the amount and fat of the same foods. If you can't drink "blue" or skim milk then change to 1% milk. It will still make a difference in the total calorie you consume.

The second key to eating control is to learn to eat SENSITIVELY. Notice that I said sensitively, not sensibly. In the general scheme of things, there are three fuel nutrients, four if you count alcohol, and we will in a future chapter, but for right now, there are three major fuel nutrients. That means we don't get calories from any of the vitamins or minerals, or from water. We only get energy in the form of calories form carbohydrate, protein, or fat. Carbohydrate and protein have the same number of calories per gram of the substance, or 4 calories per gram. But fat is over twice as effective at providing us with energy or calories. It provides 9 calories per gram, or over twice as many calories for the same amount of protein or carbohydrate. Then, in the previous example, when Karen was using just two small ladles, each ladle was two ounces, or four tablespoons of pure fat. Since there are 59 Calories in each tablespoon of dressing, and the dressing wasn't low calorie, then when she added two scoops or four ounces, she added eight tablespoons at 59 Calories per tablespoon or four hundred and seventy-two Calories to her salad. In two recent review articles, a well known physician and a researcher who specialize in the study of obesity concluded that obesity is primarily a problem of the amount of energy contributed by FAT... and not that contributed by carbohydrates and protein. They further stated that there is evidence that each macronutrient (i.e. fats, carbohydrates, and protein) is regulated separately in relation to amount eaten and total body stores. (Nutrition Reviews 45:33, 1987; Clin. Nutr. 2(2):15, 1987. Fat intake seems to promote fat storage. If this is true, then a higher protein, lower fat diet where more of the calories are made up from protein and unprocessed carbohydrate will promote better weight control. If you figure in the energy equation, that it takes three thousand five hundred Calories (3500) to make one pound of ugly body fat, then in just seven days of overindulging 500 extra Calories, or in one week's time you could have accumulated 3500 Calories, or enough Calories to make one pound of utterly disgusting body fat. Bottom line, by controlling the portion size of the fats, those sneaky calories, Karen was able to begin to reduce her weight much more easily. You, just like Karen, can learn to control your portion size of the concentrated calories, and those are the ones that matter. You do not need to go on a diet that you will ultimately go off of... and regain the weight. You only need to manage your intake and know that you are ingesting. By exerting control, you can learn to become slim. But first you have to know which portions count. And not only which portions count but which kind of calories count. For example, the calories from carbohydrates and protein do not make as much difference as fat calories. Now, this does not mean that you should eat only "fat free" foods because usually these foods have been processed and are manipulated by adding more carbohydrates or this is not an acceptable food substitute. Always choose the least processed food. The business of controlling your calories should be redefined! Controlling fat, sugar, and in general calories, should be taught just like reading or writing in grammar school, but we were not. How can you add the numbers if you don't know what the numbers are? How can you cut out the calories if you don't know where they are? Karen, just like about 88% of the people who have come to me for counselling, and instruction was intelligent, concerned, and totally ignorant of the number of calories in the very foods that were causing her the problem with her weight. She was never taught the energy equation in school, or from her parents. Nutrition was not one of the three R's in school, yet she was expected to maintain her weight when she had no idea how many calories she needed to maintain that weight, and as her body's need for calories declined she was expected to just "know" that she should eat less. Eat less in this, the bread basket of the world? We have been given an endless supply of checks, and no one bothered to tell us that at some point that supply would run out. No one expects you to keep your checking account, or your bank account balanced, without full knowledge of the amount in the account. And no one should expect you to keep your calorie bank balanced without some information on the number of calories that you need spend either. In the beginning of every session with my patients, I ask "how many calories do you need to eat in a day to maintain your weight?" The number of answers I get is extraordinary! No wonder 66 % of the population is overweight. We, as Americans, have calorie checking accounts that are overdrawn and no one has bothered to send us a letter of reprimand, or a reminder, or fine us for an overdraft, or give us a three day quit or pay rent…until the inevitable health reminder. We are among the lucky ones if we see ourselves in the mirror and think this is not acceptable. If we wait for the stroke, or the heart attack, then it's too late. Then the consequences become apparent; diabetes, cardiovascular problems, renal insufficiency or worst… a coronary occlusion; stroke or heart attack is our first or possibly final signal.

Regulation of food intake begins with you. There was and still exists in some cultures a status value of obesity. Ethnic food habits and food ways are inherited in the culture. Our American holidays revolve around our sweet tooth. Santa Claus fills our stockings with candy. The Easter bunny brings chocolate eggs, jelly beans, and marshmallow chicks. Halloween spells trick or treating when goblins knick on doors and demands more sweets. Birthday parties focus on birthday cake and ice cream. These traditions reinforce the sweet tooth conspiracy.

Avoid the problems and obstacles that are getting you sidetracked. Do not by dietetic beverages, drink water instead of soda. Use less sugar and drink your coffee and tea black or with only a bit of Stevia. Out of sight, out of mind works. So get the cookies out of sight or better yet, out of the house. Do not put the cookies in a cookie jar that screams "COOKIES" from across the room. Decide what you need, then, get the things done that will lead you closer to your goal. Know what will satisfy you personally. The world today, and ten years from now, we will continue to face multitudinous stresses in various forms every day. Monitor your stress level and determine exactly what the stress is in the situation. It probably isn't the baby crying, or your teenager asking to go to who knows where. Look deeper. Is it the bill in the mail confirming that you will not be able to take that vacation after all? Is it the phone call from your husband sharing his frustration over a work situation, or a missed opportunity for that promotion? It is usually not the most obvious irritant. It may take some searching. Then, use your assertiveness to become more effective in dealing with the problematic situation. Habits are changeable because they are learned behaviors. Pavlov's dog salivated when the bell rang. It was learned behavior. Maybe you are conditioned too, by your environment, by the clock, by the billboards, by a commercial. If that is true, you can find another way to drive home so you won't have to pass the convenience store or the bakery. Look past or around the billboard that tells you "the burgers are better..." Avoid the temptations. Don't fight with yourself when you are confronted with them. Use the same psychology that you use with your children because after all, it may very well be the child in you that is demanding the instant gratification. If the children want to go swimming, and you have firmly told them "no", do you then drive them by the lake so they can see the crystal clear water, and feel the cooling breeze?

Don't let the little things annoy you. If you are balancing your checkbook, and you pen runs out of ink, do you stop? You simply delay your task, while you find another pen but you will eventually get it done if it is tied to your survival. Sadly, I have seen too many people get discouraged about a set back in weight management. The pen running out of ink is an obstacle, a minor set back. If you are following weight conscious principles, and because of an unavoidable change of plans you find yourself in a pizza parlor with friends instead of eating a brown bag lunch it's not the end of the world. But for too many people it's the "end of their diet". The excuses begin. "Oh. I was so bad…" I really "blew" it. Then the guilt starts. "I'm no good anyway." "I'll never do it." "I just can't control myself." Think about that pen running out of ink. That's life. Remember you can shift into second gear just as easily as you can shift into reverse. You will continue to go forward, just not a rapidly. Choose to eat one piece of pizza. Choose the vegetarian option. Avoid the high fat pepperoni and have a glass of cold water instead of the soda. Doing something is always better than doing nothing at all. Whatever you do don't give up on all the hard work and successes you have had so easily. Never give up the ship.

Avoid discouragement. You meant to follow your meal pattern. You meant to exercise. You meant to park farther from the store and walk across the parking lot. But the party, the holiday, the celebration came up. Your husband lost his job. Your son got a ticket for using his cell phone. Your daughter got a promotion. You tried, but you had a very good excuse for not following through. Don't mentally beat yourself up for any of these excuses. Welcome to the human race. Life is full of surprises. Deal with the surprise, the pen running out of ink, and then get back on track. Now stop feeling guilty! Sure you enjoyed the social situation, but stop the guilt. You can simply continue with your plan. Don't degrade yourself. You've lost five pounds or fifty! That is something you can be proud of. Always count your accomplishments. You have to decide what you will now do to finally achieve your objective. First, be certain it is your objective and not someone else's goal. What will give you the most satisfaction, and what do you need? Then when you hit those inevitable I have to have a candy bar days, you can think of the pen. It's a temporary set back and certainly not the straw that will break the camel's back. It is not the thing that will stop you from reaching the most important goal you have set for your good health.

Always keep your prime objective foremost in your mind's eye. Do you really want to lose those fifty pounds or do you just want to get out of your present uncomfortable situation? Are you aiming for a healthy weight or do you just want applause from the peanut gallery? Are you craving more self esteem, or better health? Or are you simply looking for something to complain about? Is being overweight just one more reason to berate yourself for something you think you should have achieved already? Avoid the self pity. Keep yourself riveted to what you have set as your prime objective, and no matter how many times you fall of the horse, and how many hoops you have to jump through, remember you can do it if you think you can.

Increase your effectiveness with intermediate goals. Keep your healthy weight management a top priority by setting goals that are easy to achieve. Instead of ten pounds how about five. Instead of walking up three flights of stairs, how about walking up one and walking down three flights. By developing habits you won't even have to think about them once you have developed that habit. It takes thirteen weeks, before it becomes second nature. So get started today. If it is really important to your survival, it gets done. No matter how many more important issues arise in your life, getting your healthy weight under control must rank in the top three. Never forget that. Now set your intermediate goals. You have most probably been managing your life by using intermediate goals for some time. For example, you have lists, or notes around the house or office. Call to stop the paper. Get plan tickets. Arrange for the children's lessons. Stop the mail. These are all intermediate goals. It breaks down the larger goals into manageable steps, so that you can accomplish your goal. So write your intermediate goals down. Then, when you've met your intermediate goal, remember to set another one. Become goal oriented.

Accentuate the positive. Is weight loss all that counts? The answer must be "NO". You need to begin to think positively about yourself. You can do it and you can if you think you can. Remember to keep a positive self image, and the belief in the power that you personally hold the key to permanent weight reduction and management. Use booster sessions for reinforcement. Follow these keys until you have the power of any self destructive mood swings. Those are the little devils that say you can't. You must continue to believe that this change is beneficial to your health. Learn to accept eating patterns that help you arrive at the goal you want. If you eat one meal a day, your body will be in a feast or fast state. Our body is programmed to survive. More, fat is an active organ to insure our survival. If we eat essentially one meal a day, our body will become very efficient at utilizing those calories to be certain we survive. We will eat too much, too fast. If we eat several times a day our body is better able to manage the nutrients, and we will never be so hungry that we will eat anything that isn't nailed down. If you cannot eliminate something negative find a way to put a positive spin on it. For example, you simply detest the idea of going to a gym and doing aerobic exercise fifteen minutes four times a week, but on a hot day, a swim in the pool is the easiest way to cool off and oh by the way swimming laps will actually burn more calories than aerobics. Or may be you enjoy dancing. Try Zumba. That is fun and is also an aerobic exercise. When all is said and done, you are the one who is responsible for your weight state. You can pay to join a club or you can do it inexpensively with a bicycle, a pool, a video tape, walking, jogging, roller skating. Not only are these activities inexpensive, you are starting habits that will last a lifetime.

Socioeconomic class influences obesity and its development as well. Studies indicate that at the lowest socioeconomic level there is an increase in less expensive calories from starchy, high carbohydrate, high fat foods. Flour, bread, noodles, rice are the foods that are the least expensive. Foods that represent high quality protein foods are expensive, as are fresh fruits, and vegetables. This dictates what the food dollar will be spent on. Social mobility increases and the incidence of obesity decreases. The lowest socioeconomic class has over eighteen times the obesity of those who are upwardly mobile.

Advertising and other food promotions bring new foods to our attention, and influences our choices in countless and subtle ways. It is difficult to measure the impact of advertisement on our food choices. But it is significant. Advertisements may even encourage overeating. It prompts overweight or people with diabetes to buy "special" dietetic foods that are often more expensive and unnecessary. Colorful and beautifully photographed foods create a desire for specific foods. We are constantly exposed to this with the television, the internet, magazines, supermarket advertisements, billboards and more.

Feelings around foods originated with the origin of man. People ate to survive. Because of the intimate ties to survival of the fittest symbolic feelings of food arose. Many food habits are deeply entrenched with a long history of family tradition. Almost everyone has a group of traditional customs. Do you cook greens with bacon fat, or use sour cream on blintzes? These are high fat habits. Food habits continue to be the sum of our experiences with food. The clean plate club has been overdone. To some parents, a fat child is a healthy child. To some, wasting food is sinful. If you don't eat your vegetables you can't have dessert. Eat your food, because some child in a third world country is starving. We would be better off if we simply served smaller portions instead of eating after we are already full. If you have been exposed to such pressures growing up remember that significant others have placed a distorted view of the place of food in your life. This can lead to overeating, overweight and disease.

People expressed their successes and well being with excess poundage. The tribal chieftains were usually overweight as an expression of their bountiful stores. It was a societal indication that they were well and successful enough not to want for food in their homes. Even today, in the third world countries, the tribal chieftains may be rotund as an indication of good fortune, wealth and ability to provide. In more developed countries this is carried over in the form of status foods, lobster, caviar, Filet Mignon, fine wines, and champagne, or Cognac.

During infancy, we see the symbolic meanings of food developing. The infant has its first encounter with suckling at the breast, or bottle offered by someone who cuddles and hugs the baby. Here emotions become bound to the feeding encounter and associated with security as the baby is cuddled. Security and trust become entwined with food. We are satisfied. But, it is not just the procurement of nutrients needed for survival, health, growth, and development. Even in infancy, food develops its connection with love.

Further evidence of this connection is pointed out in an acute care setting of the hospital where during illness; stress is compounded in a strange and sterile environment. The child or adult patient often regresses to an earlier developmental level in such a situation searching for security. Children previously weaned from the bottle may refuse to drink from the cup or may demand a straw with liquids. Children who have never sucked their thumbs may begin to suck. Or the child who is well able to feed himself from a developmental point will suddenly need to be fed. These are all common instances and a normal expression of a search for increased security associated with eating.

Once we have identified the behavior in a child, then it is easier to make the connection in adulthood. Once again, you need only look at the hospital admission for an adult. The fully mature adult becomes a finicky eater. He demands that his egg be cooked precisely as requested, and that his toast be warm and browned exactly as he demands. Intellectually, he knows that he is one of many to be fed, but emotionally, he is demanding, in a way very similar to an infant, that his foods and he are special. He is making a statement that foods satisfy his psyche, as well as his stomach. The patient is asking for someone to care for his needs, and to send love on his dinner tray. Food is undoubtedly more than just something to eat. It is true that the role of food in our social life may be a contributing factor to overweight. We comfort our friends with candy and fruit. We thank our hostess with a box of sweets. We welcome guests with a tasteful dinner, that may be high in fat and Calories too. We exchange recipes, as a compliment to the creator of that special dish. Now, let's begin to separate food from love and begin to control our own destiny.

Eating is often a chain reaction prompted by the environment and food cues. The situation, as you saw in the hospital often dictates the mood. Break the chain that leads to overeating or eating out of stress by appropriate planning. Postpone "stress" hunger pangs by using diversionary activities with a couple of simple rules. First, the diversionary activity must be easily accessible and the activity must be in direct conflict with eating. For example, you could not use taking a rowboat ride as an activity unless you had ready access to a boat. Food is not love. Don't program it into your life as such. When you get hungry what can you do?

Use pleasant activities. For example you could include shopping, reading, sewing, or even talking to a friend. Necessary activities can also be used. For example, you may pay bills, or clean out a closet. You can also use activities for specific situations, for example jump rope, or go for a walk outside. When you are tempted to eat when you are not hungry, first know the signals and second do something else. After all, you have better things to do.

Identify problem behaviors as the first step in breaking the problem chain. Now answer the following questions honestly and candidly.

1. How much control do you have in your home environment? In your work environment?
2. Do you generally eat in one specific location?

3. Does this specific location have other distractions such as the radio, or television?
4. Do you eat slowly or are you generally in a hurry?
5. Do you have a full glass of water with other beverages at your meals?

The more familiar you are with your routine behaviors, the easier it will be to have power in your world. You can then control and change the things that need changing one step at a time as you trickle down in your weight.

Take time now to identify some of the things that you are doing routinely to make your weight management permanent.

POSITIVE BEHAVIORS:

1.
2.
3.

Now list three behaviors that need to change.

1.
2.
3.

List one thing that you can do to change the behaviors that need changing.

1.
2.
3.

You have been eating where? Engineering a Skinny Environment Checklist

When you eat be aware of what you are eating, and where you are. Make a list of areas where you should be eating and stick to those areas. Avoid areas that appear to be a problem when you discover you are eating mindlessly without regard to what you are eating.

DAY	1	2	3	4	5	6	7
Watching television while snacking							
Sitting on the patio and eating chips or a candy bar							
Drinking a soda or juice just to relax							
Eating a snack at a sports event while observing							
Eating a snack while driving your automobile							
Eating leftovers while cleaning up after a meal							
Nibbling on a snack while waiting for a friend to call							
Drinking another drink even if you are not hungry to be social							
Getting up at night and having a midnight snack because you can't sleep							
Ordering another appetizer at the bar because your table isn't ready							
Eating with friends at a pizza restaurant because "everyone was going"							
Eating an ice cream with friends because someone mentioned your weight							
Eating because you are bored							

Learn the difference between physical, situational and emotional hunger.

The only reason you should eat is because you are physically hungry. Your goal is to eat to live not live to eat.

When you need more support go to <u>www.notimefordiets.com</u>

Chapter 5

Activity A Look at the Master Stroke De-stressing Your World with Body Movement

Before beginning any exercise program, check with your physician to determine what is safe for you.

How active are you?

"Oh, I walk all day long at work. You reply.

"Gee. I'm going all day." Since your view of activity will vary so radically from one individual to another, it is important to get a baseline of where you are now. One of the best ways to measure that is to get a pedometer. That is objective and will give you an idea of where you are starting from. The goal is 10,000 steps a day. Okay, does that sound outrageous? Could you accomplish 3,500 steps by noon, 3,500 steps by 5pm and 3,000 steps by 9 PM? One thing is certain, if you are not losing weight now, and you are "going all day long", either you will need a longer day, you will need to increase the number of steps that you are currently taking during the day, or increase the intensity. Don't kid yourself. I can't remember the last time I mowed the lower forty. Can you? We don't do as much manual labor as we used to, no matter how tired you are at the end of your day.

"Why exercise?" you say. "Why not just starve myself and get it over with?" Remember that one aspect of the equation is to eliminate the negative. If you can't eliminate the negative, then introduce a positive aspect into the equation. Okay, so you really detest aerobic exercise for fifteen minutes four times a week, how do you feel about a swim in a cool pool on a hot day, just to cool off? Gotcha! That could easily be transformed into the fifteen minutes of aerobic exercise, with a fun twist! Once you are in the pool, before you begin your leisurely paddle, get into the water chest deep and run form one side of the pool to the other. This will work well for those who are only slightly overweight as well as those who are obese. Running in the water cushions and lessened the absolute weight and pressure that you would normally be placing on your knees when you walk. The labor savers we enjoy today are important considerations in our failure to get enough exercise daily. Under present conditions, many children as well as more adults have very low levels of energy expenditure. How many times have we driven the children around the block when they could very well have walked? Or count the times you have jumped into the car to get something at the convenience store down the street, just one or two blocks. Inactivity contributes significantly to the development of obesity. Obesity is a matter of energy balance. Many people have a plan that hasn't worked well in the past. As activity increases you caloric intake tends to decrease. With advancing age, our basal metabolic rate decreases which means we use even less energy to do the essentials like breathing. Couple this with decreased energy expenditure of today's labor saving inventions of modernization, and you have the recipe for obesity.

According to research in the American Journal of Clinical Nutrition, (24:1405, 1971) during caloric restriction the amount of energy that is needed, that is resting energy expenditure declines significantly. Therefore, dieters are encouraged to increase their physical activity to compensate. Aerobic activity increases the resting energy expenditure in persons undergoing moderate caloric restriction defined as 1200-1800kcal/day. We have long known that exercise helps lose fat. According to the International Journal on Obesity 9:39, 1985 and the American Journal of Clinical Nutrition 46:622, 1987, exercise does appear to promote the loss of fat rather than muscle. And that, my friends is exactly what we want to achieve! Keep the lean mass and lose the ugly fat. A reducing regime will work far more effectively if used in conjunction with a moderately increased physical activity program, which has been specifically planned with your specifications. To lose weight you must either take in less Calories than you need, or burn up more Calories than you take in.

"I don't have enough time now!" The hectic schedule is a call to make some time for you. If you are experiencing the "no time to say, hello, good-bye…I'm late I'm late I'm late" syndrome. Then exercise in your personal world is just what you need.

Successful weight management involves more than just eating less. Sedentary people often have an increased appetite that is not related to the lack of activity. With those people who are moderately active, the increase in appetite is closely proportional to their energy needs. This is according to a study by Meyer related to West Bengal workers. As our activity has decreased with modernization, its importance in the energy equation cannot be underscored. We must bring our energy expenditure to a level where our body will recognize and regulate our food intake with energy output. Compare your Calorie intake with energy expenditure to see how you are doing. Remember to reduce, you will need to take in 500 Calories than you use in a single day. Create a deficit of 3,500 Calories in one week, and one pound of body fat will disappear.

Activity can help accomplish some of your personal goals too, not only of weight management, but also of dealing with and decreasing stress. Body movement reduces stress. These practices take a little time but will help give you the feeling of improvement and a measure of success. Exercise will give you the control, and the realization that you yourself are reaching the specific goals you seek. Exercise will give you the control and realization that YES, you are worth the effort and YES you are succeeding. Good habits fuel the fire that you have begun. You don't have to join a health club. A health club will provide some measure of weight loss in luxury for a price. However, when all is said and done, you are the person who is responsible for your own weight state. You can pay to join a club or a spa, but you can also accomplish the same goal inexpensively with your own bicycle, or a pool, walking, jogging and controlling your own intake. Now only is this method free, it's free for life! Jog two miles a day, or swim laps in a pool to get the activity to help your new body look its best. But before you start, be certain that you set a specific goal with a specific aim in mind. Have more than a general idea of what is going to be involved. Know what will be specifically required in your planning. See yourself reaching that goal, and perhaps more importantly, see the specifics of when, where, and how you will reach it. You realize that activity and increasing energy output are of prime importance in the development of healthy weight, now; you will want to find ways to fit this into your new healthy lifestyle.

"Won't that would be even more time away from my family?" Not necessarily.

You can accomplish your secondary goal by increasing family time as well. The relationship between physical activity, weight control and maintenance is now becoming increasingly emphasized in successful formulas for weight management. For instance, regular exercise can prevent the development of love handles and potbellies characteristic of middle aged men. Without exercise, the average thirty-five year old man will gain nearly one half to one and a half pounds of fat each year until the age of sixty. We are composed for striated tissue known as fat; essential fat that cushions our vital organs and protects them form shock and trauma, such as the fat pads surrounding kidneys.

Additionally, we have the fat free tissue, or lean body mass, which is comprised of the muscle and bone. Your internal chemistry then, is the sum of the adipose tissue metabolism, and lean body mass metabolism, plus individual difference.

Research seems to indicate that the fat body mass can be differentiated into two types of fat; brown fat mass, a faster burning mass, and white fat, a slow burning, storage mass. Both types of fat burn fewer calories per minute than the lean body mass or muscle mass. It follows that the more fat tissue that you have, very simply, the less calories that you burn per volume.

For example, if there were two men who were identical in all physical aspects except the amount of body fat, they would burn calories at different rates. Sam, with 27% body fat, and John, with 18% body fat, although identical in all other aspects will not need the same number of calories to maintain their respective weights. John will actually burn more calories just lying in bed than Sam will. Why? Because lean body mass burns calories faster than fat does.

Can you change that? Sam could minimize the difference by regular exercise. You can too! Remember, fat is overly proficient at storing energy. That's its job! It is much less proficient at burning energy or calories. Secondly, over fatness or obesity has a hobbling effect. The actual movements in our daily life will require more effort since it takes more calories to move a larger mass from one point to another. The body compensates by becoming more efficient, and will make less movement. If you doubt this, watch an over fat person, and a thin person jogging, or even walking. Which person makes the most movement in getting from one point to another?

Increasing your energy output can be accomplished without joining a gym or spa. You can park your car farther away from your building, and walk across the parking lot. Walk to the door of the building or office and then take the stair rather than the elevators. Walk the stairs and use the elevators only as a last resort. If you can't walk up all twenty flights, then walk up ten, or five, or start with two or one. Gradually work to increase this. You can't spare the time you say? Are you in too much in a hurry? How much time do you want to donate to your good health? How much time do you want to spend with your grandchildren? How important is a healthy lifestyle. And how much of your retirement do you want to spend in the hospital? A brisk walk upstairs, or across the parking lot will improve your cardiovascular system, and burn unwanted Calories as well. It will help realign your internal chemistry. And, after all, who cares about being a model. They have their problems too. Wouldn't you rather be a model of health?

A young patient of mine proved the theory that one size does not fit all in lifestyle activity only too well. This adolescent and her mother both came into my office and although the adolescent was referred to me, the mother, who was also overweight, insisted on coming as well. Being a somewhat dominant woman, she took a great deal of the time away from my counseling with her daughter. Session after session, we set goals that were mutually decided upon, but for the daughter, these met with limited success. He mother was about to give up when I suggested that she might want to wait in the waiting room while Carol and I met. The mother agreed reluctantly. Carol confided that she was being overwhelmed by the goals that her mother was imposing upon her. I insisted that Carol should only work on the goals that she felt she wanted to and felt she could accomplish. The next session, Carol came in and weighed two pounds less. This trend continued for several more sessions. Finally, the mother was invited to sit in on the session. She was astonished to find that Carol had lost twenty-four pounds. Her mother, who had remained the same weight, exclaimed, almost in dismay,

"How could she have lost that weight? We are eating the same things."

Carol confided that she had been getting off the school bus one stop before her house and walking the extra six blocks to her home. That was something Carol could do. She had set her goal and had found a way to change her lifestyle to accomplish that goal. She had increased her activity to get the exercise that she hadn't been getting. That is what made the difference.

Finally, sedentary people have more time to eat than those who are moderately active do. If you increase you daily activity, you will have less time to eat. Our modern lifestyle with its stresses and sedentary patterns coupled with individual inactivity lends itself to the "Let George Do It" syndrome. Emotional needs that arise between your food and your mouth contribute to your self-image. If, for instance, during developmental stages, you're physically awkward, to avoid the ridicule of your peers, you may tend to follow a pattern of less physical activity. You'll tend to stay from the embarrassing or painful situations. Our search for peer acceptance teaches to avoid activity where we might not display our best qualities. We sit out of the game or cheer the team rather than partaking in sports which would use up those Calories. Worse, we munch on a hotdog and soda while we watch. Ever notice how much food and beverage is consumed while watching the Sunday football games?

To compound the problem, our own self-image progressively deteriorates as we store more empty calories in our fat deposit bank. Personal and social stimuli act to develop this image from early childhood. The Super Heroes and Super Heroines are classic, svelte, athletic figures. The fashion models have stick thin figures. Oralness that we have developed in suckling too, may contribute to overeating, for example, buying an ice cream to lick, or sucking on a straw. The long, tall refreshing lime Ricky or mint julep that we sip on adds its toll without even a clue that there are in excess of one hundred empty calories in each glass.

Once you admit that activity and increasing energy output are of prime importance in the development of normal weight, your next thought will be,

"But with my life, there's no time left for exercise."

Let me share a few ways that you can increase your energy output.

77

1. Parking your car at the farther space away from your office building or store, or doctor's appointment and walk to the door of the office or store.
2. Walk upstairs, and use the elevators only as a last resort. If not twenty flights, why not ten, or two or one. Gradually work to increase this.
3. You can't spare the time, you say? Too much in a hurry?

How much time can you donate to your well being? How important is your life?

How important is your health? A brisk walk will improve your cardiovascular function as well as burn unwanted calories. Surprisingly, exercise will actually increase your basal metabolic rate. That is the rate that you burn Calories for internal functions. For example, the energy it takes to make your heart pump blood to your vital organs, the work of breathing, and the energy to make your kidneys, pancreas, liver and all the other organs function.

How active are you?

"Oh, I walk all day long at work." You will probably reply.

Or, "Gee, I'm going all day."

Since activity levels vary so radically, from one individual to another, and are usually decreased with this modern day society, it's important to have a baseline for your own individual physical expenditure. You know that you are not losing weight with whatever amount of activity that you get during the day now. Then, you should concentrate on increasing your activity above your present level. According to research in the American Journal of Clinical Nutrition (24:1405, 1971) during caloric restriction the amount of energy that is needed, that is the resting energy expenditure, declines significantly. Therefore, dieters must increase their physical activity to compensate. Aerobic exercise does increase the resting energy expenditure in persons undergoing moderate caloric restriction (1200-1800kcal/day), according to the International Journal on Obesity (9:39. 1985). Further, the American Journal of Clinical Nutrition 46:622, 1987 suggests that exercise does appear to promote the loss of fat, rather than muscle, and that, my friends it exactly what we want to achieve.

For the person who takes up exercise for weight loss the goals of exercise are tailored to meet your goals. If you take in the number of calories that you burn up you will maintain your weight. To lose one pound of body fat, you will need to take in fewer Calories than you burn up or burn more Calories than you take in a day. If you have a Calorie deficit daily of 500 Calories than at the end of one week, you will have a deficit of 3,500 Calories or one pound of fat.

For the most effective weight management program you should choose activities that require at lease 5 kcal/min and use approximately 300 calories per exercise session. The exercise should be performed at least three and preferably four times weekly. At the same time, the caloric intake should be reduced but not to a point where good nutrition is compromised.

Keep the lean mass, and lose the ugly fat. An effective global weight management program with commitment to a moderately increased physical activity program spells success. To lose weight, you must either take in fewer calories than you need, or exercise to burn up more calories than you eat. If you eat less and exercise more, the results will be twice as satisfying. If you have a Calorie deficit of five hundred calories each day for seven days, then at the end of one week, you will have a deficit of 3,500 calories, or one pound of body fat. Further, if you exercise within two hours of eating, more kilocalories may be burned off than if you exercise on an empty stomach according to research published in the Journal of the American Dietetic Association, 83:3:290, 1983. This makes the timing of exercise important. If you exercise after eating you stimulate the metabolic rate; the rate at which calories are burned. This same research supports the idea that the heaviest meals should be eaten at breakfast and lunch since most people are more active early in the day. The intensity of the exercise is not as important as the regularity of the program. Sedentary people often have an increased appetite that is not related to increasing activity to a certain point. With those in the moderate activity category, their increase in appetite and intake in closely proportional to energy needs. This is according to Meyer in a study on West Bengal workers. Since our activity levels are decreased with modernization, it's important to bring our energy expenditure up to a level where it is easier for our bodies to regulate our food intake with energy expenditure. Compare your calorie intake with your routine expenditures in one day to find out how you are doing with the Calorie equation. To reduce, you can create a deficit of 500 calories a day, and in seven days create a deficit of 3,500 calories, or one pound of body fat. Further, if you exercise within two hours of eating, more kilocalories will be burned off than if yo9u exercise on an empty stomach according to research published in the Journal of the American Dietetic Association, 83:3:290, 1983. This makes the timing of exercise more important. Exercising after eating stimulates your metabolic rate, the rate at which calories are burned. This same research supports the idea that the heaviest meal should be eaten at breakfast and lunch since most people are more active early in the day. Do you remember the old wives' tales that advised to eat like a king at breakfast, a queen at lunch and a princess at dinner? Those old wives may have had something there. The intensity of exercise is not as important as the regularity of the program.

You've decided to do it! Congratulations. Start by limbering up exercises. Stand with your feet apart, and stretch to touch your toes. The most important exercise of any physical fitness program is the warm up. These prepare the muscles and body for a more strenuous effort at exercise. These exercises should be done until you feel the effect. A proper warm up will work up a bit of perspiration, but not tire you out.

1. Arm Circles: Holding arms out to the side at shoulder level, with palms up, circle forward, then backward with palms down, ten times.

2. Shoulder rotations; with arms hanging loosely at the sides, circle shoulders forward then backwards, five times

3. Knee lifts; standing pull right knee to the chest, return right foot to the floor, and repeat with the left leg. Repeat this five times.

4. Trunk twisting; Stand, hands clasped behind your head, twist trunk laterally, first to the right then the left, ten times.

5. Vertical arm lifts; Standing, arms at sides, lift arms straight up in front and over head twenty times.

6. Lateral arm lifts; standing arms at sides lift arms out to side and up overhead ten times

7. Side Bends: Standing hands clasped behind head bend at waist, side to side. Repeat ten times.

8. Head turns; Turn head; side to side fifteen repetitions.

9. Bent knee sit-ups: Lying on floor, on your back, knees bent flat hands clasped, move to a sitting position and back. Repeat ten times.

10. Abdomen Exercise: Lying on floor. Slightly bend one leg. Raise other leg straight up as high as possible keeping the knee straight. Lower raised leg slowly until it is three inches from floor, and hold it for ten seconds. Release and repeat with other leg. Repeat five times.

11. Hip and thigh exercise: Begin on hands and knees. Balancing yourself with your hands, lift right leg up behind you with knee straight. Lift it up and in an upside v motion. Repeat five times. Change to left leg and repeat five times.

12. Pelvic tilt: Flatten back by squeezing buttocks together, and tightening abdominal muscles so that your pelvis tilts forward. Avoid raising or pushing feet.

13. Partial sit-up; Begin with pelvic tilt position. Tuck chin and curl shoulders and back as far forward as possible, forward towards a sitting position. Hold and uncurl slowly to the starting position.

Since none of these exercises require a great many Calories to perform, they should not be a substitute for the exercise sessions that would be classified as aerobic. These exercises will aid in toning your body, and should be done a minimum of three times per week. Always start slowly when attempting new exercise activity. Be careful not to overdo. You can always increase your exercise capacity a little bit at a time until you reach a good exercise level that is vigorous but not too strenuous.

Now that you have decided to exercise to help with that weight loss, you will no doubt want to know what type of exercise will most beneficial in terms of both burning calories, and conditioning our cardiovascular system. Your body weight is constantly changing, with growth, maintenance, and repair. During weight loss, it's important to burn up the fat stores, yet avoid the starvation, and stress which tend to burn up the lean body mass. People, who engage in only intermittent, non-strenuous sports such as the weekly game of golf, or doubles tennis, may be kidding themselves if they think that they are reducing the risk of heart attack. They should be asking the question, fit for what? The answer might be; your unhealthy de-conditioned lifestyle. You don't have to be athletic to be fit. You don't have to be a long distance runner, or an Olympiad. The exercise prescription should include frequency, intensity, time and type of exercise. If you can't do it all at first, don't be discouraged. No one expects you to. Again just use the principles routinely and continue to build on your successes. Those who expend a minimum of two thousand calories a week in physical exertion, have, according to research, significantly fewer heart attacks (64%fewer) than those who expend fewer calories. Activities that burn the most

Calories include walking, jogging, swimming, bicycling, skiing, and hiking. Too, it should be noted that if you are significantly overweight, it might be wise to begin your exercise program with a running underwater type of exercise. Since the water acts as a cushion, there is not so much of an insult to your knees, and will decrease injuries that you might sustain to the feet, or knees when putting too much pressure during exercise. Adjust your program to five days or as few as four days per week. Remember, to maintain your present state of fitness, participate three days a week, to improve cardiovascular conditioning, increase your activities to four days each week. Try to skip every other day or at least do a different activity to give the muscles time to recover. Now that we have two thousand Calories as a goal, how do you expend those Calories? There are several ways to accomplish this.

Walk four miles in an hour five or six times a week.

Play forty-five minutes to an hour of singles tennis five times a week.

Ride a bicycle 45-60 minutes average eleven miles an hour, five times a week.

Alternatively, bicycle twelve miles an hour, four times a week.

Jog at a five-mile an hour pace for an hour three or four times a week.

Increase your speed to six miles an hour and jog three times a week.

Other exercises are just as beneficial. For example jump rope for twelve minutes. Run in place, stepping over chairs. Work for fifteen minutes jogging, cross-country skiing, rowing, dancing. Use a mini-trampoline for fifteen minutes. Exercise for twenty minutes walking, bicycling, ice skating, roller skating, or swimming. What ever type of exercise you choose to do, **DO IT ROUTINELY.**

Finally, think fun. Dancing can be great exercise and can expand your social life. These exercises and team sports can be a great way to expand your social life or improve your relationship with your family. Kids love to go to the zoo or any of a variety of theme parks where there is plenty of room to walk, and run.

Two other side benefits to regular exercise of any type are that it increases the HDL, the body's "good cholesterol" and it will increase your production of endorphins. Endorphins are a group of polypeptides in the brain that raise the body's threshold for pain. These hormones behave like opiates. Endorphins may help you to deal with stress, pain and menstrual discomfort and provide increased appetite control, too. To derive the maximum benefit from your exercise program, attempt to achieve this goal. Raise your pulse rate from its resting rate to a target rate and maintain that rate for twelve to fifteen minutes. This means that you are pushing your heart harder to do its work. You are over exerting rather than conditioning it.

To find your pulse rate sit quietly in a chair.

Place your index finger and third finger on the side of your Adam's apple.

Count the number of beats for fifteen seconds. _____

Now multiply that by four. (X 4) = _____

(Average Pulse Rate = 70-80).

To figure your target pulse rate subtract your age from 220.

220 – (your age) =_____

Multiply that by .70-.85_____

For example, say that a 30 year old had a pulse rate of 60. His exercise target rate would be 160. What these figures mean is that during your exercise session, you want to raise your pulse rate to your target rate and keep it at that rate for twelve or fifteen minutes. You are exercising at 70-85% of your maximum. Take your pulse for fifteen seconds and multiply by four. Is it up to your target? No? Then work a little harder as long as you feel well. If it is over what you set as your target, then slow up and cool down. You don't want to exceed your target. If you exceed your target that means that you are stressing your heart unnecessarily. Ten minutes after you have stopped all movement, take your rate again. It should be back to your resting rate. You've done a good job, and you can congratulate yourself on that.

The degree of enthusiasm with which you undertake any exercise, will also have a direct bearing upon the Calories expended in the activity. Remember the quote by Ralph Waldo Emerson. "Enthusiasm is one of the most powerful engines of success. When you do a thing, do it with all your might. Put your whole soul into it. Stamp it with your personality... Nothing great was ever accomplished without enthusiasm." If you think this is just another "ho-hum cure-all" rethink your mind set. Think of the child who races back and forth across the room and the frustrated adult who chases him. Aside from the fact that the child's metabolism is higher, that child is running with the enthusiasm of life, and in so doing will burn fat more calories because of the amount of enthusiasm that he shows for "the game". Learn from the child inside of you. Get on the Exercise bicycle with a smile and a zest for a healthy lifestyle. Don't put it off until tomorrow. Tomorrow may never come. Do it today. Activity lifestyles can be learned behaviors too, and you can change them and help to increase your health quotient and permanent weight loss. Forget about letting George do it. Get up and do it yourself.

Recommended reading: Fit or Fat, Covert Bailey, Houghton-Mifflin, 1978

Chapter 6

Work Place Wonders: Power on the Job

In our hectic, "No time to say, Hello. Good bye. I'm late I'm late. I'm late" world it's important to know not only what you intend to accomplish but what got you where you are in the first place. In the workplace more often than not, external cues may tell us that you "need to eat". More frequently than not, our lifestyle at work will reinforce this external cue to eat.

At work, breaks from work are frequently associated with food. The ten o'clock break may have coffee and donuts, or bagels. Lunchtime is usually the same time. Everyone takes a break from work and usually eats something. The clock on the wall reaches twelve and as boredom for the current task takes over; you glance up at the clock and your stomach growls. You may think of the vending machine, or the cafeteria, or the shop down the street, and decide that it is time to take a break with friends and the "comfort from the work routine". Or perhaps the person next to you opens his or her lunch box and the aroma of a barbequed chicken sandwich, or the treat from McDonald's waifs through the air. You have been tempted by external cues. Or perhaps a work mate goes to the vending machine and returns with a mouthwatering Three Musketeers or a small bagful of your favorite fresh roasted peanuts. When you see this tempting treat, voila! You are "hungry" for a little something. You have just been lured by external cues to eat. Your next action is often automatic. You probably never stop to think what that little something costs in terms of fat, or total calories in your energy account.

"It's lunchtime, isn't it?"

"You have to eat, don't you?"

The answer to both of those questions is yes, but have you considered if you are really overspending on your calorie account? It's a shame that like credit cards, we are not presented with a bill for the calories we have spent at the end of every month, or every week, or even in one day. Unfortunately, if you are like many Americans, you are in debt and close to or over your credit limit. So, too, you are over extended in your energy account. Even if you *have* learned to control the amount of money you can spend, few of us have stopped to learn exactly how many calories we can spend to gain, lose or maintain our weight.

What we need to know, besides how to balance a checking account is how to manage our energy account before we are hopelessly overdrawn. In a society where there is virtually no physical activity needed to exist, the normal physiological control of our energy balance may be faulty. When you respond to external cues, you are responding to stimuli rather than the true physiological hunger. Instead of responding to the stimuli, be certain that what dictates eating is physical hunger. To be certain that you know how many times you reach for a nibble, or a snack, or a meal of break with food involved during the day, during your work week, and on the week-ends use the "When do I eat?" chart. For this exercise, it's not important to write what you ate. Just place a check at the time that you ate. This will help you identify how many times you actually ate during the day, and evening. It will help isolate multiple or chain eating periods, as well as pinpoint particularly dangerous times.

Where do you eat? Most of us eat because we are in a situation that triggers our appetite, senses and brain. Possibly, we may eat when we find ourselves in a boring or stressful situation. We may have also trained ourselves to eat when we are depressed or angry or frustrated. In fact, any positive or negative emotional situation can cause the emotional animal in us to be released. Many foods are considered reward foods, fetish foods, and showoff or status foods. For example, whipped cream, lobster, or a lollipop all connote some of the emotions just described. Many people may not be able to distinguish physiological hunger from other states such as fear, anger, or anxiety. You can even illicit a response which may fool you into having gastric sensations. When in an emotionally charged state, you may salivate, have dry mouth, and feel weakness, irritability, or nervousness. This super sensitivity to signals visually is directed by environmental cues.

Boredom, frustration, and low self esteem can increase the urge to eat or inappropriate eating. Emotions then, tip off the eating response rather than physical hunger. Do you know people who can be categorized as a nibbler, a binger, a sneaker, or a prowler? These are all emotional eaters. Social conditioning has given us a model. If then you change food availability you can build cues to control and monitor you behaviors. Then use contingency management and find out where you need to make changes. Using the checklist for when you eat, begin to notice where as well. Especially take note when you find yourself eating. When you are at work, eat in one area only. The same can apply when you are at home. When you eat, only eat. Avoid other activities, especially avoid turning on the television. It dissipates your thoughts and before you know it you may be responding to an advertisement for some snack that would have been better if left untouched.

Why do you eat? A block or conflict keeps us from achieving your goal. This frustration causes our expectations and desires to change. This makes it difficult to deal with the new demands and causes adjustment demands. For example, a boring job, however uneventful it may be turns out to be the least demanding. Even common frustrations such as delays related to traffic, or life in general, may **be** psychological blocks. Other frustrations more closely associated with stress are loneliness, losses or failure. Different people have different strategies for approaching a conflict. You may approach-avoid, approach-approach, or avoid-avoid. The closer we get to our initial goals, the better other goals look. If we approach the problem of over fatness, we will increase the stress in our lives. As the stress becomes more overwhelming we are less likely to carry through with our log term goal of decreasing our fatness. Although increasing importance of the goal will increase the stress we feel, also the longer you work to accomplish a goal, the more stress you will feel if it is unresolved. Adding several goals at once will also increase the stress. Stress is increased if we are unfamiliar with the goal or we anticipate the stress of a particular goal. This is particularly problematic when the goal is weight loss because many times we use food as a panacea, a solution to our problems, or a security blanket. When we are unable to use food we must find another solution, and a way to deal with difficult situations. Set your boundaries. But remember that it's okay if you find you want to change your boundaries. When you identify your challenges, and then is the time to begin the task of retraining yourself. Use imagery to adapt to a possible situation where you have had less than ideal control. Imagine yourself saying, "No!" Take personal time out to work through any obstacles. Always give yourself the choice of two or more solutions. Practice "what if" scenarios. Change from reactive to active and set behavior goals. Decide on a solution and mentally act it out. Would you propose that course of action with a history similar to yours? Then, work out your coping behaviors. Be patient and do not over extend yourself. Avoid guilt. But analyze, and revise old behaviors and ideas. What behaviors are getting you sidetracked? Decide what it is you need. Then get the things done that will lead you closer to the larger long term goal.

Diets don't work indefinitely. The main reason is because at some point, you will "go off the diet". You will begin to feel guilty for "breaking the diet". You will feel sorry for yourself because you couldn't follow it, and the weight will unfortunately return. But now you can change the tendency to "be overweight." You have the power to change your life pattern. You can change your eating habits and your body image because you now have the knowledge and the power to do it and be successful at this without going through the deprivation syndrome.

Diets are only a temporary change in your normal eating pattern. They foster a state of mind of sacrifice. This is not a winner's attitude. It is not the attitude that will help you to maintain your weight loss and continue to lose weight to your initial target weight and your final weight goal. It is nor is it the way to learn heart healthy eating patterns or incorporate activity patterns that will ensure you continue to be at your cardiovascular best. Any kind of austerity pattern will help you maintain your weight loss only temporarily. Unless you make permanent changes you will go back to your original eating habits; the ones that caused you to become overweight in the first place.

The more you know about yourself, the more you can effectively control the Calories and the environment that you find yourself eating and drinking in. No place can be more telling than the workplace. This, despite our best efforts is where we are apt to spend most of our time. These are the people who become our significant others, our friends, and unwittingly, our therapists. These people had better be good because for many of us these are the people to whom we confide our most private dreams, thoughts and fears.

At some point you will need to bring your weight reduction efforts to your workplace environment, and see if there is a fit. Successful weight reduction and understanding the fundamentals of good nutrition are imperative. This is because after reading this book, you are most likely, unless there is a registered dietitian in your midst, to be the best informed about weight management principles and control.

Habits are changeable because they are essentially learned behaviors. Pavlov's dog salivated when the bell rang. That was a learned response. You are most probably conditioned by your environment, by the clock, by the billboard, by the commercial, and these conditioned responses can be unlearned.

The first challenge is to identify the areas, and people in your workplace that have provided you with learned responses that involve food. For example, when someone brings in candy or bagels or other treats are you one of the first to partake? Remember, eating should be a conscious act rather than a habit or the result of some emotional response such as boredom or fear. Be kind to yourself. You have already decided that you are worth the effort and can and will be successful in this effort. You need to take care of yourself. Don't save the special perks and grooming for a special occasion. Those don't come along frequently enough. Instead when you are relaxing, relax only without the benefit of food. Use a swimming pool or a spa or Jacuzzi. Take an oil bath, or give yourself a facial, do you nails or any other kind of personal indulgence you are particularly fond of. This is the most important self acknowledgement. You are succeeding and you know you are worth it. Do it just for the health of it. Finally, develop your own support system. A successful healthy lifestyle is one that you become, not one that you try. Make it fun, and develop a mutually supportive system of colleagues. Family and friends are in many cases able to support you as well as help themselves to lose that evasive few pounds. It is always easier to do if you know someone is supporting your efforts. You want to win. You want to develop a lower resting pulse rate and increase your fitness and improve your health. Then, use your pattern and with the help of your friends, develop a healthy lifestyle. Use problem solving, and find ways to avoid difficult times, but don't do too much too soon.

You're ready! Get set! Set a goal! Make it one that's easy and one that you cannot fail to achieve. It must be something simple. It can be as small as a substitution. Words of caution here in goal setting for change; never make the change for more than a week. This period is manageable, and more manageable than next month. A lot can happen even in a day! Maybe one pound may sound miniscule, bet remember, that involves avoiding or burning 3500 Calories! Too, because the time is short, you will need other indicators of your success. Avoid only five hundred calories you would otherwise have eaten, for one day! Decide to do it each morning when you are getting ready to start your day. Don't start tomorrow! Tomorrow is just a dream. Don't count on your successes for yesterday. That's history. Decide to do it for the health of it for a finite period of time, not a week, not a month or a year. Simply decide to do it for one day...today!

Successful weight management means understanding the fundamentals of good nutrition and continued good health hinges upon understanding food composition and the body's use of food that are ingested. As you begin to take this program into the work place, take the time to answer this simple quiz to see how well you understand nutrition and the principles of weight management. It's a simple true and false quiz. The answers are at the end of the quiz.

1. Dietetic food should be used anyone who is trying to lose weight?
2. When a label on a food product reads 'Light" that means that the product is half as fattening as the original product or replacement counterpart.
3. Honey is allowed on a reduction pattern because it is a natural food and as such it will not contribute the same calories as sugar.
4. Sugar has as many calories as margarine.
5. Grapefruit melts away fat, therefore it is essential on any reduction diet.
6. Alcohol has fewer calories than sugar.
7. It is a good idea o fast occasionally during the weight reduction pattern.

8. Potatoes and bread should be avoided on any reduction pattern.
9. Gelatin is nonfattening and will help grow fingernails because it is high in protein.
10. When trying to lose weight, it is best to eat one meal a day.
11. Older adults need fewer nutrients than a twenty-five year old adult.
12. Polyunsaturated, no cholesterol means less calories.\
13. Margarine has fewer Calories than butter.
14. Yogurt and cottage cheese have been shown to help with weight loss and can be eaten in unlimited quantities on a weight loss pattern.

Now the envelope, please.

1. FALSE. Dietetic implies that the food has been modified in some way. The modification may simply be the omission of salt. Dietetic does not necessarily mean low calorie. Nor does it mean that is especially suitable for a diabetic.
2. FALSE. Light simply means that the manufacturer modified the product to provide 25% less calories than the original food. If the original food was a very high calorie product to begin with, the "light" version, with only 25% less calories may also be a high calorie product.
3. FALSE. Honey is produced by bees and hence is a natural product, to be sure, but it does not have any fewer calories than sugar. As far as added nutrients, the nutrients in honey contribute an insignificant value. Honey's major contribution is still calories.
4. FALSE. Sugar is a disaccharide, a simple carbohydrate. All carbohydrates provide 4 Calories per gram of carbohydrate. Margarine is a fat. Fat is a more concentrated source of Calories, contributing 9 Calories for every gram. Then, margarine gram for gram has more than twice as many Calories.
5. FALSE. No one food, whether grapefruit, papaya, or green beans will magically melt fat away...unfortunately.
6. FALSE. Alcohol yields 7 Calories per gram, thus compared to sugar at 4 Calories per gram, sugar is less calorically dense than alcohol.

7. FALSE. Fasting can actually reduce you basal metabolism, effectively causing your body to burn less calories.

8. FALSE. Potatoes and bread are two unjustly maligned foods. They provide important B complex vitamins, and are not particularly high in calories. Instead, limit the extra fats, like margarine, butter or sour cream that tend to accompany the potatoes, and bread. And be careful to avoid the concentrated carbohydrates that don't contribute much except calories like candy and regular soda.

9. Gelatin does contain calories and is an incomplete protein, and there is no evidence that gelatin alone will help fingernails grow.

10. FALSE. Gorgers, those that eat one large meal actually utilize the food more efficiently than those who graze, or eat several smaller meals during the day.

11. FALSE. Older adults need the same number of nutrients as young adults. In fact, because of the less efficient absorption of some nutrients, an older adult may need more. Only the number of calories required decreases as we age.

12. FALSE. Polyunsaturated fat has the same number of calories as a saturated fat such as butter has. Just because the food has no cholesterol that doesn't necessarily mean it is low in calories.

13. FALSE. Margarine has the same number of calories as butter. Only the type of fat is different. Margarine is a polyunsaturated fat. Butter is a saturated fat. Diets high in saturated fats have been linked to heart disease. However, margarine in a manufacturing process called hydrogenation can have the polyunsaturated fat hydrogenated (or hardened) making a trans fat, which is utilized by the body like a saturated fat.

14. FALSE. Any food will add to the total calorie intake, and no food can be eaten in unlimited quantities without it affecting the total. A cautionary word about yogurt, many of the brands may say fat free or low fat but have extra sugars added. The added sugars boost the calories making the food a high calorie treat.

To assess what you are doing most effectively, put time and distance between your food choices. Before you even get out of bed, think about what you want to start off the day with, and make an informed choice.

If you decide to take those extra few minutes to catch up on your beauty rest, consider this. You have heard it! Breakfast is the most important meal of the day. Studies have shown that the meal in the morning assists in the increase in midmorning efficiency. It will also help you resist that office coffee break when Kathy brings in Dunkin Donuts. So, begin each day with breakfast. Include a good source of protein, like some low fat cottage cheese, egg whites, plain yogurt, or a glass of skim milk. Add cereal and fresh fruit. If you have a piece of whole wheat toast or an English muffin, use fat only to taste sparingly. Don't forget, the fats are the sneaky calories. Warm toast spread with butter or margarine easily melts and can add up to unwanted pounds. Be careful, too of concentrated sweets such as jam and jelly and other dental caries producers. They are not contributing nutrients in any significance except calories. If you do decide to have jam or jelly those will count as part of your discretionary allowance for the day. When you decide on a bagel instead of the toast, know that you are choosing a high calorie food. One bagel can easily add an additional 350 Calories to your once skinny breakfast. That's not even counting the cream cheese!

Chapter 7

"I'm Late…I'm Late…Meals in a Rush"

Armed with the best of intentions is never enough. When you are in a crunch for time or money either time or money will win out over the best intentions to keep on track with healthy food. For example, without planning what your plans are for the next twenty four hours, life will generally take care of that for you. No, it's not exactly what you think. You will wake up, but too late to have a sensible breakfast, and then maybe just a cup of coffee, or worse you can stop at Starbuck's on the way to work and pick up a Frappachino and maybe bacon, avocado egg wrap. Those muffins look great and it's easy to carry while driving and texting on your way down the freeway. When you get to the office, someone has been considerate enough to have stopped and picked up some donuts that look wonderful, and the office pot of coffee is hot and you are ready for a refill while you plan your workday. There are some leftover See's candies that someone sent to the office to tell the staff how thankful you have been for your services. Someone's child has had a birthday over the weekend and the parent was thoughtful enough to bring in the leftover cake. It is chocolate layered with whipped cream and certainly worth taking at least one bite. Well two more cups of coffee should help to get your creative juices flowing and the workday world is in full swing. Everyone has to talk with everyone about what went on since yesterday and then finally, there is time for some work. Coffee break is coming up. Then there is lunch, which you have forgotten to think about. Someone in the office is going out to the Mexican restaurant, or a fast food stop off, and they are more than happy to pick up something for you. By midafternoon you are beginning to feel a bit tired, and you cannot understand why. Could be you haven't really fueled your body with anything except caffeine, fast food, high fat, high sugary treats and your body would benefit from some "real food". As the workday world continues to unfold, there are deadlines, and you begin to think that you could eat nearly anything that isn't nailed down. You determine that you will need to have a "good meal" at supper tonight. That "good meal" is yet to be determined and when a friend calls and invites you to supper at the Cheesecake Factory to just get caught up on old times; it sounds like the chance to have the meal you haven't eaten all day. Whew! Well maybe all this isn't packed into every single day but its representative of more than a few. And that is the real issue. You can follow that disjointed schedule for a day or two but you cannot continue to hope that the day will afford you the opportunity to eat a healthy meal plan unless you have some sort of schedule or structure in mind first. There are a wide variety of delectable foods readily available to tempt us. Restaurants from fast food to fine dining have all joined the super size revolution. It's an established fact that a proper diet plays a major role in your good health and successful weight management. Unfortunately, unlike smoking, if you choose to quit smoking, you can use any variety of methods to change that habit. The primary consideration is to actually STOP SMOKING. You can live without it. But if you want to lose weight, you cannot simply stop eating! What you have to change is the type of food choices you have been making. You must be able to select healthy food choices in a variety of situations and this is a skill you will need to develop and use for the rest of your life. You already know that following basic nutrition guidelines makes sense, and you will develop the skills to follow these guidelines when you are buying groceries as well as preparing meals. You will learn the skill sets to manage your meals away from home, whether it is on vacation or at a business meeting. That way you can make sure you are getting the foods that not only taste good but help you to manage your weight and resize yourself to a healthy weight. But what if you are like the millions of Americans who eat out regularly? You are at work or away for home most of the day, usually eat lunch at a restaurant or grill. It is not forbidden to eat at these restaurants, but it is important that you watch what you eat on the go and be certain it fits into your meal plan. Over the years, physicians and highly specialized nutrition experts have identified key parts of the diet for staying healthy. Experts in nutrition have used this information to look at the food value of the menu items listed. Nutrition guidelines for the fast lane help you identify exactly what you are getting in that super sized meal. There are three basic guidelines for good nutrition that can apply to everyone. First, eat a balanced diet. That phrase does not simply imply one that will not fall off the plate. It implies instead that you eat a variety of foods to provide the known nutrients in the correct quantity for health. Choose foods that are low in fat especially lower in saturated fats, and that the fats you choose are the "healthy" fats, those being the unsaturated or monounsaturated fats that are heart protective. These fats are high in EPA, and DHA, and have a good amount of omega-3 fatty acids. Finally, avoid foods that are highly processed and overloaded with sodium. In ancient times salt was a valuable item and was actually used as a means of monetary trade. Eventually it became an inexpensive preservative. Today, manufacturers understand the importance of sodium. Food preference for higher sodium foods is learned, and consumers will purchase foods higher in sodium because of personal preference. The problem with sodium is not that it's a learned flavor response. Sodium is a mineral that can cause our vessels to constrict. Sodium in and of its self can cause vessels to become more rigid. If you think of our vessels as a hose that initially is flexible, then our heart the ultimate pump pushes blood through our vessels and they flex. As the vessels become more rigid, and flex less these vessels as more inflexible and resistant to the force of the blood as the heart pumps it to our organs. Then you will understand that as the pressure increases against a more rigid vessel, our blood pressure tends to increase. If our goal is to keep our vessels flexible then we need to think about the amount of sodium we want to consume to keep our vessels able to flex. A good goal for your blood pressure is less than 130/80.

Often people think that eating fast food means you have to settle for foods loaded with calories, and fat with limited food value. Today, as manufacturers realize consumers are becoming more nutritionally literate, these very restaurants are modifying their menus to accommodate the more sophisticated consumer. After all, the fast food industry started for one reason; to make a profit in a changing world. They did not care what your weight, cholesterol, blood pressure or general health was. They cared that you could purchase a product they provided. They learned to accommodate consumers who were beginning to have two adults working. There was less time to prepare food at home and less inclination to raise produce, or to tend a garden. What you need to know is what you are getting in terms of fuel nutrients. When restaurants offer a sixteen-ounce sirloin, they are providing you with 975 Calories, 45 grams of total fat and 112 grams of protein. That one serving of steak provides the RDI (Recommended Daily Intake) of protein for a two hundred and fifty pound person. It provides twice the RDI for cholesterol for any person and nearly half of the Calories needed in an entire day. Fast food restaurants are past masters of the Super Size Revolution. Today, you can benefit from the government regulations that require major restaurant chains to provide nutrition information similar to that found on the labels of the food you buy in the supermarkets.

Buffets and salad bars urge patrons to have "all you can eat" for one set price. Sadly we have been convinced that its "okay" to gorge ourselves in such places because is would be a waste of time or a shame to pass up such a great deal. How many times have you eaten dessert not because you were still hungry, but because it "came with the meal" or it just looked too good to say no to?

Let's rerun to the beginning. It's late when you get up. Maybe it's too late for a sensible breakfast, but what's wrong with taking some plain yogurt, covering it with blueberries, strawberries, grapes or other fruit in season? Okay, maybe yogurt or granola or other portable breakfast are too healthy for you...what about just a hardboiled egg and a piece of bread and peanut butter? That is portable, and if you don't want to hard boil eggs yourself, you can buy them already hardboiled. Voila! You have a high protein breakfast and healthy food for the fast lane. Take it with you. But do not stop and pick it up on the way. No matter how healthy the food service establishments make it sound...its not! Eat your portable breakfast at work when you are organizing your day. And while you are organizing your day, it might not be a bad plan to think into the future as far as tomorrow so your plan will be more in place. Plan your day and work your plan makes sense for work and food intake as well. Someone said breakfast is the most important meal, maybe it was your mother. And as you know, mothers are always right! The reason she is right, and the research backs her up on this is that breakfast is literally breaking your fast. Theoretically, you haven't been eating anything since last night. (Well, maybe that's not really true, but we will talk about that later.) For now, trust your mother. That higher protein beginning, since it will take you longer to digest, will allow you to forgo the high sugar, high fat snacks at the office and will help your teeth to be less inundated with high sugar and the opportunity to build plaque, as well as maybe helping those dendrites in your brain to focus on the task at hand (that being your work). Remember, what you eat today, will walk and talk tomorrow. The food we eat is both a source of fuel to provide the energy including body heat and metabolism internally as well as externally for muscle activity and work. The food we eat also provides a source of nutrients for the continual repair and maintenance of all tissues. All foods can provide fuel for energy. There are three fuel nutrients if you do not count alcohol. Carbohydrate is the body's preferred source of energy. It can raise your blood sugar more than any of the other nutrients. Carbohydrate comes from starches, and sugars. The natural carbohydrates such as those found in unprocessed fruits, and vegetables have a lower glycemic index and will affect your blood sugar the least. The problem occurs when these carbohydrates are processed. The fiber is broken down. As the fiber is broken down the starch which is a polysaccharide (many sugars) is broken into a form that our bodies can digest. Cows can digest grasses because they have three stomachs. Since we only have one stomach, if we eat seeds or grains that contain fiber that has not been cooked or processed, we cannot digest these starches and they help bulk up our stools, but we do not benefit from the extra calories they would provide. The carbohydrates added during processing such as corn syrup, processed wheat are all available to us as additional calories. For example, if you look at an apple, applesauce and apple juice, you will see we cannot digest the skin or seeds, we eat this food slowly and it provides a lower glycemic index, but good satiety value. If we eat a serving of applesauce, most of calories from that apple are available to us. Finally if we drink apple juice, you can drink this very rapidly. There is no fiber so virtually all of the calories are available to us and quickly. It will raise our blood sugar very quickly. If you have a juicer take a few apples and find out how many apples you will need to use to produce ½ cup of apple juice. You may be surprised.

Protein is the fuel nutrient that is the body's building blocks, and is needed for growth, repair and maintenance. Unlike carbohydrate, there is no storage for protein in the body. Amino acids are the building blocks of protein. There are twenty odd amino acids in nature. However, we don't need to eat all twenty amino acids. Our amazing body can make nearly all of the twenty amino acids by various combinations as long as we get the eight or nine essential amino acids from the food we eat. These eight or nine amino acids are called essential because it is essential that we get these amino acids from our diet. For infants and rats there are nine essential amino acids, for the rest of us there are eight that are required to be obtained from the diet. Beans, nuts meats, fish and dairy products are good sources of protein. Both protein and carbohydrate provide four calories per gram for our energy needs.

Fat is the final fuel nutrient. It insulates the body, and cushions and protects vital internal organs. Fat provides nine calories per gram and comes from sources such as olive oil, butter, animal fats such as the marbling in meats, the skin in poultry, and dairy products. No one food provides all the essential nutrients. We therefore need a balanced diet of different foods. Most foods are a mixture of protein, carbohydrate, and fat along with varying amounts of vitamins, and minerals.

Chapter 8

Supermarket Survival; What labels Don't Tell You

Make it your business to know portion sizes and control them. During a busy day at work with no time for lunch, I sometimes buy a pint of milk for my lunch. As I stepped up to the counter one day, with my carton of milk the clerk mentioned something about Calories. I told her I was trying to increase my Calories.

She said, "That's not high in calories."

I mentioned that it was 300 calories.

She said," No, it isn't." She pointed to the carton which said 150 calories per serving.

"That's true, "I said, but there are two servings in a container, and I'll drink the whole thing." That's something she hadn't thought about. It's important to read labels, and then translate what they tell you. You see, she had read the label, but then she hadn't applied the knowledge to the container size. Be careful with labels. They tell us something and we need to know what it is that they tell us, but what they DON'T TELL US, is even more important!

The nutrition information on the food labels should tell the consumer what the product is, honestly and accurately. If the product is enriched, that is a particular nutrient that may have been destroyed in the processing is added back to the product. For example bread is enriched with thiamin, riboflavin and niacin. If a product is fortified, specific nutrients are added that were not originally in the product. An example of this is orange juice fortified with calcium, or milk with Vitamin D. The label must give the name, place of manufacturer, packager and distributor. It must not have a misleading container size, and is required to states the addition of any artificial color, chemicals and preservatives. The name must be displayed are the common or usual name, in accurate and simple terms. The listed ingredients must be in order of the largest first to the smallest. The labeling standards are structured to tell you nutrients in the food, and any nutrition claims. It will tell the serving size, and the number of calories per serving. It will also tell you the number of servings approximately in the container. This is important, because you want to be certain of the number of calories you are eating. All labels have a standard format, but the serving size is not standard and can be adjusted by the manufacturer. Optional information may also be provided on various nutrients. With the newer labeling regulations, potassium will soon be required and in the future, hopefully phosphorus may be required as well. There are advantages to nutrition labeling since it makes it easier for you to compare products and evaluate the nutritional information. It has raised the nutrition consciousness of both the food industry and the consumer. However, the labels may give the consumer a false sense of security and there are no regulations to identify whether or not the food is genetically modified. Foods can be fortified from 50% to 150% of the RDI (Recommended Dietary Intake) with supplements. Fortification over 150% of the RDI is considered drugs. Some foods are exempt although they have nutrients added, for example iodized salt, and foods with nutrients added for technical reasons are exempt. An example of this is the use of ascorbic acid (Vitamin C), or phosphorus when used as a preservative, or stabilizer.

Planning ahead for meals forces you to become more aware of what you are eating. It helps you obtain nutritious and appealing meals to compliment your healthy weight program. There is no safe formula or safe short cut or miracle methods to take off unwanted pounds. In planning your purchases, buy healthy meats, fish and poultry. Skinning the poultry will remove about twenty calories or more per serving. All cuts of meat should be trimmed of fat, poultry skinned. Never have more than 15% fat in any cut of meat and use chuck arm roast, flank steak, filet mignon, sirloin roast steak or tips, tenderloin, round and rump of all cuts. Use leg of lamb, or loin lamb chops, trimmed, pork loin, leg and all cuts of veal. Again, remember all poultry should have the skin removed. It should be broiled, roasted, without the addition of high fat ingredients. Keep seafood in mind since most all seafood can be highly recommended. Broiled fish is satisfying when sprinkled with paprika, chives, and lemon and garnished with parsley. Add a sliced sweet onion when broiling fish in foil, for a slight change in flavor. Avoid frying and limit extra fats, sugar and flour when possible.

Use Teflon coated pans, or skillets for browning, and use non stick spray of olive oil. Use a metal rack when broiling or roasting to allow fat to drip away from the meat. As the meat cooks, basting will season the meats. Low calorie marinades can bring fresh and interesting flavors to your creations. Use lemon juice, tomato juice, soy sauce, and Tabasco sauce for flavors. Pour the marinade over the meat, and use a plastic bag to close it. Press the bag to distribute the marinade. When you are making gravy place drippings in the freezer briefly, the fat will rise to the top and can be removed easily.

The portion size of your entrée is best no more than 5-6 ounces. Livers are highly nutritious, but also high in cholesterol. You can safely eat livers once or twice a month. Soups are delicious on a cold evening. Make them with broth or skim or 1% low fat milk. Other good seasonings for meat and vegetables are chili powder, Worcestershire sauce, A-1 Sauce, horseradish, capers, mustard, garlic, onion, curry, chives, green onion, vinegars, both seasoned rice wine, and apple cider vinegar. Read the labels when you buy spices and avoid the seasonings that have salt listed in the ingredients. For example use garlic powder, or onion powder rather than garlic salt or onion salt. Use wines to flavor, but avoid "cooking wines" since they are higher in sodium. Instead use table wines to enhance. When thinking about sour cream, a tasty lower calorie substitute is low fat cottage cheese, blenderized, or plain low fat yogurt. Either of these can be used when making party dips. When selecting cheese it is important to use the lower fat choices. Aim for fewer than 10% fat or under. Some of these choices include part skim mozzarella, parmesan, Romano, farmer's or pot cheese, Weight Watcher's, or Chef's Delight.

Waterless cooking allows fresh vegetables to cook in their own natural juices, thus both conserving the nutrients and flavor. Seasonings can be added to the vegetables before or after cooking. Microwave cookery for vegetables works well. Substitute herbs, vinegar and lemon juice and limit the butter and olive oil to keep the fat calories to a minimum. Remember, that the fats contribute more than twice the calories gram for gram that carbohydrate or proteins do. Retain the low calorie benefit of salads by tossing the crisped greens with lemon juice or vinegar. Make tomato cups to hold salad mixture. Cut off the tomato top and scoop out the pulp with a spoon. Turn the tomatoes cut upside down on absorbent paper towels to drain before stuffing. Chop the pulp and use in the salad.

Serve sandwiches open faced to eliminate the second slice of bread. Softened margarine spreads more easily so less is needed to cover the bread. Remember to be stingy with fats. To reduce calories from beverages for punches and fruit drinks use sparkling water, or low calorie beverages. Just before serving pour carbonated beverages down the side of the bowl or pitcher, or use a freezer tray to freeze low calorie ices. When the mixture is frozen break with a fork. For whipped ices transfer chunks to a chilled bowl, and beat until smooth. You can use Kool Aid and instead of using sugar try Stevia.

Plan to serve one food in each meal that can be eaten in essentially unlimited amounts such as lettuce, celery, mushrooms, cucumbers, peppers, radishes, cabbage, broccoli, and cauliflower, in fact, nearly any vegetable. Uncooked vegetables are higher in fiber and so provide more satiety value at the end of the meal. For your workplace preplan by bringing you own emergency supply of cottage cheese, tuna, hard boiled eggs, and the like for breakfast and lunch. Remember, any recipe can be made "diet" if you avoid frying and read the ingredients. Then look for ways to reduce the amount of added sugars, cut the fat in the recipe, or change the type of cheese to a lower fat variety. Substitute lower fat milk for cream or fat free cream cheese. Use marinades for spice.

It's easy to be overwhelmed with the barrage of advertisements that claim miracle weight loss. Our automated society gets work done rapidly and without pain. We want the same magic for our weight loss and weight management. But remember that everyday you will exert full control over some aspect of your life. Use a shopping list to avoid sabotaging yourself when you enter the market. It might be beneficial to make a quick shopping guide prior to going to the store. Write specific brands if necessary. These would include staples to have on hand when planning is less than perfect. Use this as a guide to choose and enjoy the foods that are both healthy and good for you. Remember these simple tips before you go shopping. Never shop on an empty stomach. Before you go shopping EAT! Make a physical list. By this I mean, not just a mental list of the foods you will need in the store. Avoid the impulse to buy snack items. Stick to the basics until you are sure how many "extras" you can safely handle and still lose weight. Shop when you are not in a hurry and do so infrequently. The more often you shop the more nonessential items you tend to buy. From a financial standpoint just remember, don't eat much and you will always have enough. Shop at the same grocery store routinely. Then, organize your list according to the aisles in the grocery store. Only go down the aisles that you need to. You can organize the coupons by aisles too. When you enter the store go around the outside of the store. That is where you will find the produce, cheeses, and dairy products.

Every day there are things that are not in as much control with our eating habits as we would like. To break this pattern, for a few days, make it your business to know portion sizes, of everything that goes into your mouth. Once you know how much you are eating, it's easier to decide to have a different size portion, and allow yourself to have larger portions of the high fiber, low calorie foods without feeling any guilt about eating it. That gives you a greater feeling of control. Often, clients will say, I just cannot control what I eat when I am entertaining business contacts. Become familiar with the common household measures for your meals, particularly the teaspoon and the tablespoon. Learn how much your handful will hold. To learn how much **your** handful will hold. Take an ordinary household cup measure and portion out the following; measure 8 ounces of water. Now pour that amount of water into your favorite cup or mug. Does it hold more or less than eight ounces? Then pour four ounces of water into a juice glass that you would typically use for orange juice or other juice. Did you know that the accepted serving size for a glass of juice is four ounces? The amount of liquid you drink becomes more important the more calories or sodium that it contains. For example, tomato juice although low in Calories, will cause you to have more fluid retention. It may cause problems if you are taking any medications for high blood pressure. A lower sodium intake will help antihypertensive medications work more efficiently. If you are actively losing weight, and are eating a higher sodium diet, in many instances fluid retention may mask an actual fat weight loss. Decrease foods that are particularly high in sodium such as soups, or high sodium juices. Any foods that are high in salt or high sodium mask actual weight loss. So if you are actively watching your weight loss and you do not see the scales move, decrease the salt in your diet. Do not use any added salt in cooking or at the table, whether regular table salt, sea salt or kosher salt. Instead use Mrs. DASH, herbs, spices, or other salt substitute that does not have "salt" in the title or in the list of ingredients. There are over two thousand milligrams of sodium in one teaspoon of table salt. Limit the total sodium intake for the day to less than two thousand milligrams. This way you are eliminating any possible obstacles that could discourage you and get in the way of your success. In general, begin to read labels and get a postal or other digital scale. They are relatively inexpensive. This will measure ounces or grams. Then the next time you are preparing dinner, weigh out ounce of meat. Examine that amount closely. Not much is it? Then add meat to it to provide three ounces. That is a serving size! Take a piece of deli lunch meat and weigh out an ounce. Weigh a chicken leg with the bone. Now remove the bone from it and weigh the poultry. Know that over ninety percent of the fat in poultry is in the skin, and the dark meat has more calories from fat then the white meat. Skin your chicken or turkey. Go to the freezer and look at the meats, chicken and fish that you have purchased. Look at the total eight in pounds and ounces that you have purchased. Using a three or four ounce portion, how many portions will that total weight of meat, chicken or fish serve? If you are allowing more than a four or five ounce portion per serving, that is probably more than you need, and you have just added extra unneeded calories to each meal. This is especially true if you are serving meats, such as beef that are highly marbled. Finally, compare this size of portion to the portions served in the restaurant. What a difference! Now it may make more sense to you to ask for a "doggie bag" for half of that meal before you begin your meal out. That way you can sanely eat out and enjoy a second meal "out" at home. Give yourself the praise that you deserve for the number of changes you are making and the changes with the types and amount of foods that you are consuming in one day. For example, did you know that merely by switching form regular soda to water, for every twelve ounces you would be saving approximately one hundred fifty calories or more? One of my patients at Redondo Beach

Medical Clinic proved that fact resoundingly. She came to my office weighing over two hundred pounds. At five feet tall she would have been considered to have clinically severe obesity for her height. She was a mother of three young children and spent many hours daily with them. She had an advanced college degree and had chosen to spend time raising her children. However, the work of motherhood, although essential and always challenging is not particularly taxing mentally a good deal of the time. To ease the boredom, the mother read and while she read, she consumed Pepsi Cola. During a typical day, when she filled out her food diary she noted that she drank three or four Pepsis a day. When researching the portion size what was remarkable, is that these were two Liter containers. She was unwittingly consuming three thousand five hundred and ten calories each day from the Pepsis alone. When she became aware of her error, she was able to substitute water and lose weight quickly. She did this by literally eliminate enough Calories from the soda to lose one pound of fat in one day! Just a word of caution about changing from a high caffeine beverage to a caffeine free beverage; there is a potential for caffeine withdrawal. There is a need to distinguish between habitual and no habitual users, and moderate and excessive use. Most of the pharmacologic effects of caffeine result from the AMP catabolism cycle. Oral intake of caffeine is absorbed with peak plasma levels occurring within fifteen to forty five minutes. The caffeine in cola drinks is metabolized more slowly perhaps because of the lower temperature, and acid levels, and the higher sugar content. Heavy users of caffeine (over one thousand milligrams daily) can produce symptoms of anxiety, dizziness, nervous irritability, insomnia, headaches, and tremors. From two thousand to four thousand milligrams can actually precipitate psychotic reactions, and aggravate psychotic process in mental illness. Headache is a common withdrawal symptom of habitual caffeine intake. Other symptoms include less alert, less active, more sleepy, more irritable, jittery, nervous and shaky. How else does caffeine affect the body? It can function as a diuretic, a mild antidepressant, an antispasmodic and an appetite suppressant. In addition, it dilates the blood vessels, and stimulates the nervous system. Caffeine may also stimulate the basal metabolism, and the action of the adrenal glands. It stimulates gastric secretions, which may irritate the stomach lining. Although some people say that their caffeine intake never interferes with their sleep pattern, most people will agree that a bedtime cup of coffee may interfere with their slumber. Both children and geriatrics are affected by caffeine to a greater extent than the adult population. Caffeine is metabolized differently in pregnant women and takes thirty times longer to be eliminated by the fetal brain. Then, how much is too much? A cardiovascular and sports nutritionist in the Boston area and author of "The Athlete's Kitchen" considers over two hundred and fifty milligrams of caffeine daily excessive. An eight ounce of brewed coffee can contain from one hundred to four hundred milligrams of caffeine, depending upon the strength, type of coffee, and method pr preparation. Perked coffee is usually weaker, and freeze dried, or instant coffee averages from fifty-five to sixty-five milligrams per cup. If you are ingesting more than 250 milligrams of caffeine per day, you might want to consider gradually decreasing the total amount of caffeine daily in your diet. Allow your body to adapt to a smaller amount of caffeine intake gradually to prevent withdrawal symptoms. How much caffeine have you had today? You might be surprised. Everyone knows that coffee contributes its share of caffeine, but teas, cola drinks, chocolate, soft candies, and puddings also contribute. Additionally, some across the counter headache and cold remedies contain caffeine as well. Don't forget to read the labels and count these.

Become a label reader. You then will be able to know exactly how many calories are contributed from each of the fuel nutrients; carbohydrate, fat and protein. Even if the label tells you only the number of grams of fat, carbohydrate, and protein per serving, you can quickly and effortlessly calculate the number contributed by each. For example, if a particular product for one serving contains 3 grams of protein, 10 grams of carbohydrate, and 12 grams of fat then by using the formula; of four calories per gram for drank carbohydrate, and protein and 9 calories per gram for at you will find that thirteen grams contributed from protein and carbohydrate is fifty-two calories and from the 12 grams of fat at nine calories per gram contribute another 108 calories, thus the total from the serving is 160 calories for the food. Read the labels and especially take note of the serving size. Often the manufacturers will adjust the serving size to make the food look more healthful. For example a Hershey's chocolate bar provides two and a half servings. Now if I could find two and a half friends of mine to share the candy bar with that would be fine. Unfortunately in this fast paced world I will likely eat the entire candy bar myself. So what started out to be a healthful treat, has become more than my fair share of discretionary calories for a snack in the middle of the day. Any cheeses made with nonfat or 1% milk are more acceptable since they have a good source of protein and the fat is limited. Take care to stick to nonfat or 1% milk especially if you are drinking this as your beverage. If you choose low fat, or 2% milk that is no real savings in fat since whole milk is usually 3% fat. The milk based beverages are naturally higher in sodium though.

Macaroni, rice and noodle products are good plain, but be careful of the gravy, sauce, and margarine that is added. Meats are great sources of protein, but be very careful of the portions allowed per person. Juices, seafood, and deli are usually on the outside of the store. Fish canned, frozen or fresh are excellent sources of nutrients, protein and healthful fat, but sadly underrated. Take care with bakery products especially with flour. 1 tablespoon goes a long way to increase calorie intake especially with breading, sauces and gravies. Look for no sugar added, and especially be aware of dried fruits. Dried fruit have the water removed, making them dangerous because they are small, portable, and an easy snack to munch several at a time without thinking they are truly whole fruit with the water removed. Remember how easy it is to eat four pears, dried without realizing that you have just consumed four hundred Calories. Honey should be used as just a sugar. It has no significant nutrient contribution even though it sounds healthier. It is truly no better than the processed table sugar, without much in the way of nutrients provided. Jams and jellies too are just another processed form of concentrated sweet, with or without the "additional sugar added" they are merely another form of concentrated sweet. They along with cookies and crackers contribute extra calories and sugar that rot your teeth. Cocoa and chocolate are frivolous items. Ice cream has too much sugar, and fat! Save this for a special occasion. Yogurt is not the dieter's dream unless you use plain, nonfat unflavored yogurt as a substitute for sour cream. It contributes one fifth the Calories.

Read the labels carefully. Dietetic foods are not always low calorie. These are not a necessity unless you feel an affinity for the large profit motive of companies bend on your dollar for a product with no significant contribution to your health, but instead a detriment to your teeth's health and a drain on your pocketbook. Do not buy treats for company in case they drop buy. You may find that you are treating yourself to the treats. Instead have family members responsible for buying the treats and storing them out of sight. Then, you will have the treats when they are needed, and not eaten thus available when you do want them for company.

When buying beverages, water is still the best dietetic drink. Beer and other alcoholic beverages should be consumed in moderation. Again, avoid routine purchases. Breads like bagels, hard rolls, and baked goods are usually higher in calories and fat. Avoid cake mixes and candies. Butter and margarine usually provide 45 Calories per tablespoon. Use ketchup and mayonnaise sparingly. Condiments including spices, mustard, vinegar, pepper, dill, and lemon are legal in all amounts. Cranberries, unsweetened can be used in unlimited amounts. Fresh fruits and vegetables are a must whether baked, broiled, broiled, steamed baked, or raw. Initially, avoid sugar coated cereals. Use cereals without added sugar and try to cut the extra sugar you use in processed foods to none. The easiest way to achieve this is by reading labels. Reading labels with frozen foods are particularly important to avoid brine packed.

As far as snacks, nuts are a quick munchable snack, if unsalted are full of healthy nutrients, but also have a good amount of fat. These calories can quickly mount up so if you eat them, you must eat one at a time and enjoy the twenty chew rule before you swallow. This might be a great time to enjoy the mouth feel of the nut or dried fruit. Roll it around in your mouth and enjoy the texture. Olives are high in fat, and although it is a good unsaturated fat, they are also high in sodium because of the processing. High sodium foods especially chips and salted snacks will cause you to drink more fluid as well as retaining it. This is especially true of soy sauce or instant or highly processed foods such as luncheon meats. But remember, salt is an acquired taste, and a learned response. Taste your food before you use the salt shaker.

Chapter 9

He Who Hesitates Loses Weight
Controlled Eating Response
and Sensitive Eating

Food is a basic need, but the way that you eat is learned. With repetition habits are formed. You receive cues that cause you to elicit an eating behavior, and these results in some type of reward. There are five w's that will help you to discover what the cues are to unconscious eating; they are what? When? Where? Who? And Why? The cue may be as innocuous as the television, the clock on the wall, your favorite chair, a particular commercial, the simple act of picking up the mail, or even the mere act of entering your home. All of the stimuli in your environment give you cues unconsciously. Facilitating stimuli make it easier for you to react by eating. For example, having enough money to buy food, and knowing how to cook it are to facilitating stimuli that reinforce eating. Instructional stimuli give you a cue such as a regular mealtime, or even the sight of food. Potentiating stimuli such as peer pressure or social reward may reinforce eating and finally discriminating stimuli such as prior learning may help you eat for reasons other than physiological hunger. Human nature being what it is if someone tells us what to do we may attempt to defend our position even before we really understand the significance of what the other person is trying to accomplish. Do we tend to stop listening before all the facts are presented? The first step is to learn the difference between true hunger and false hunger. The best way to do this is when you think you feel hungry, take a walk, call a friend, catch up on housework, or correspondence. Clean the basement, or wash your car. Never respond to what you think may be hunger at the first call. Remember in a crisis situation, almost all people will return to doing things that they are used to or find comforting. A food cue is a craving for an anticipated taste. Be aware of these. Don't let the television or internet commercials fool you. A certain food will not make you more attractive, but some commercials can be very subtle. Movies don't really represent popcorn and candy. The time of day should not be a signal "Whoops. I missed lunch." In the market your favorite foods are placed at eye level and many of the packages allow you to look through the wrappings. Stick to your list, and focus on what you need, rather than what you want because of the attractive packaging. Analyze the facts, both pro and con before deciding that breakfast is not in your future. If you decide to change rearrange your eating pattern, do so slowly. The process of change is really quite simple yet unique. It is a culmination of steps each of which has special significance. That may be one reason why behavior modification is not always successful without direction. The changes are dictated by what is significant for you to accomplish. Further, it must be significant to you, not your nutritionist, or physician, or friend, or parent… to you. But what is the significance of change? First, you must be aware that the change is beneficial for you, and that it has importance. Eating should be seen as a social behavior. Reinforce controlled eating. Eat slowly, and make yourself aware of the control you are exerting. Eat at different times to become aware of your physical hunger and differentiate it from the clock on the wall telling you its time to eat.

Remember the dinner table scene when you were ten? Close your eyes just for a minute close your eyes, and think back. Did anyone tell you, "Hurry up."? You have to get going to school. Come on, we need to go shopping. Or did you just stop for a quick bit to eat at the fast food restaurant because we just have a few minutes before we need to be who knows where. Was your family always in a rush to go somewhere?

Sensitive or mindful eating comes with not only controlling the rate of eating but also being present in the moment of eating as well. It may help you focus on the activity of eating and the associated feelings of fullness. Do you walk by the candy jar at work and mindlessly grab a chocolate, or hard candy or something else and you cannot really remember exactly what it tastes like? Take time to really savor the food, instead of concentrating on other activities such as watching the television, or checking your emails as you power through lunch. Remember that your stomach has sensor receptors that sense distension. Basic physiology is at work here and the sensors signal the brain that you are full. These receptors need approximately twenty minutes to send that message to the brain that you are full. The appetite center of the brain can be satisfied with less food by using delay techniques to increase the eating time and decrease your food consumption. If you leave the table within fifteen minutes from the time that you sat down, then you left before the signals have had time (twenty minutes) to travel up the spinal column to your brain and tell your brain, you are feeling full. If you are a fast eater, you can easily overeat before you even get the message that you are full. By then, you may be eating much more than your body needs. It will tell you…later! But then you'll feel bloated, and uncomfortable! Then, it's too late because you've eaten an excess number of calories!

Beware of accidental reinforcers. These are repeated inadvertent pairings of consequence with behavior. For example you are in a social situation; dining at your friend's home. Her mother is an exceptional cook, and has made enough food to feed a small army. You want to please your friend and compliment the family. A plate of scalloped potatoes is handed to you for the second time. She has just innocently encouraged and reinforced overeating. How do you refuse graciously? Refuse with compliments to the chef until she blushes. After the meal, compliment by helping her clear the table. After the meal a sincere hug will work miracles. You will be invited back again. According to one particular study, people may eat with their eyes as much as with their sensor receptor signals that they are full. Two groups of people were compared with bowls of soup. Group A had self filling bowls and the other group B did not have bowls of soup that continued to refill. Group A, the group with the self filling bowls ate a significantly larger amount of the soup than Group B, but did not report feeling any fuller.

At work do you try to fit all the errands you want to run, and lunch into a half an hour? Do you even remember all the things you have eaten at the all you can eat buffet? If you can eliminate the urgency to hurry, and control the rate of eating you will be able to control the amount of food that you take in. Put your fork or spoon down between bites. Remember the glass of cold water before eating any meal or snack. Chew for twenty bites before swallowing. Eliminate serving dishes from the table. Use a smaller plate to limit serving sizes that are over generous. If you are right handed, use your left hand, or use chop sticks. Control the total amount of eating and control the chewing rates. Really take time to enjoy the mouth feel of a grape or a raisin. Remember those sensors, and the time it takes the sensors to send the message from your gastric pouch up your spinal column to your satiety center. If you leave before the signals have had time (about twenty minutes) to travel up the spinal column to your brain, you may be eating much more than your body needs before you get the message that you are full. One way to overcome this is to start with a cold glass of water. Drink this eight ounce cold glass of water at the beginning of every meal or snack. This will do two things; first it will give the sensors a head start and secondly it will increase adiponectin which facilitates fat burning.

Do you routinely eat after seven in the evening? For one week make yourself a reminder to avoid snacks after 7PM. This will make you more aware of your habits and more able to modify the faulty ones. Why is eating after 7PM not such a great idea? If you equate your food intake to fueling your car, you can see why more clearly. Preplanning what you eat is related and very important to the techniques of control. If you're having difficulty, prepare your food for meals and for snacks in the morning and label them clearly. Put them aside and when snack time comes, you have a preplanned snack, in the correct portion ready to eat.

You can eliminate the urgency to hurry, and control the RATE of eating you will be able to control the AMOUNT of food that you take in. Control the eating and chewing rates. Give your body time to send you the message that you are full. Use relaxation techniques to allow a stress free time to think. Everyone needs time to relax and one of the positive aspects of activity is that it increases your endorphin levels and helps to reduce stress. The problems won't go away necessarily, but they will be in better perspective. Slow gradual change is best. It allows the learning process development. Many factors influence your normal energy balance. It may be environmental, heredity or as a result of your coping mechanisms. Respond to productivity not depression. List the cues in your environment that lead to your thoughts of food. It is important to recognize the signals when you are tempted, then do something else. Identify the links in the behavior chain, and identify where you can stop to interrupt the chain. Avoid the last three links; the urge to eat, eating and guilt. List alternate behaviors. Use your self control to follow through to your goal despite well meaning friends, and suggestions to eat just one more. Everyone enjoys company while eating; after all eating is a social event. You enjoy eating and drinking with friends, but you must know what is good for you. Love yourself and your health and improving self image. This is not a course in self deprivation; it's a lesson in self knowledge and your control. Know that you are not restricting your diet; rather you are becoming aware of what you are eating and drinking. You must remember that no matter who loves you, one person always will. That person has to be you. Count as you chew, and put down utensils after you take a bite. Control the amount you serve by using small plates. Eat half of what you plan. You're on your way to a slim body. How do you feel about that?

Chapter 10

Engineering a Skinny Environment Cognitive Restructuring and the Power of Preplanning in your World

Fears of becoming slender have caused more than one dieter to regain the weight that they have worked so diligently to take off. First decide that this is exactly what you want. Reduce concentrated sweets, reduce concentrated fats, control portion size, and increase physical activity. Use practice to retrain yourself. Habits are changeable. They are learned behaviors. Remember that the person who is overweight or obese is extremely attractive, and may be using this excess weight to advertise that they are no threat. You are saying, I may be highly intelligent but I am no threat. Please befriend me. Stop those thoughts! You need to use every physical and mental attribute that you have. We only have one choice. Just do it! You will not be less masculine, or less feminine. Many women have confided that as they lose weight their breasts will be smaller, and that will make them less feminine. The feminine body is one with curves in the right places. The svelte female body will become even more feminine and draw even more attention without excess adipose tissue that is concealing the true beauty of your form. Another fear, often expressed by males is that as they lose weight they will lose control, and will have less strength. When one of my clients was asked to draw an image of himself in his present state and a picture of himself after he had lost the excess weight. The picture of the slender self was almost childlike in size as compared to the first drawing being significantly smaller in stature and size. When asked why the two pictures were so different, he explained he would lose all his strength. You will be just a strong when you lose the extra fat. You will have more energy. You will be carrying far fewer pounds around all day long. At the end of the day you may be pleasantly surprised that you still have extra energy.

Learn the fine art of relaxing. Stress and anxiety are involved in almost any weight reduction and management plan. Simple tension release exercises slowing then tensing each part of your body can be helpful in determining whether when your body experiences the feeling of hunger that you're feeling a response to stress. Simple stress then release exercises can, many times, help the hunger related to stress feeling stop. To determine whether you are having a physical hunger or stress related feeling try a fantasy escape. Take five or ten minutes in a quiet room. Close your eyes and imagine yourself in a peaceful setting where nothing can bother or harm you. This is automatically calming. To fortify your resolve indulge in an elaborate daydream. Picture again what you will look like as your slender self, what you will be doing, and they clothes you will be wearing. Remind yourself of your short term and intermediate goals. With self confidence, you can do it. Assess your goals and be certain they are realistic. Do not overtax yourself. Use positive thoughts to their maximum. If you think you can do it, you can! When you reach these intermediate goals reward yourself perhaps with a new orchid, a new piece of clothing or an additional piece of equipment for a favorite sport or hobby. Plan an outing with your friend or family.

Now step back and impartially, analyze the facts. Analyze both the pros and cons of any change, for example breakfast in the morning or the rearrangement of your eating pattern to a three plus two schedule. The process of change is really quite simple and unique. It is in fact, a culmination of steps, each of which has special significance. What is the significance of change? There has to be significance and importance to the learner. You first must become aware of change. Then, you will ultimately weigh the advantages, and disadvantages of the prospective change. If the change advantages outweigh the disadvantages, then you will incorporate that change into your daily routine. The more you know about yourself, the more effective control you can exert over your environment and the efficient control of the Calories you find yourself eating and drinking. Give careful consideration to your habits and how they have been formed.

A number of interactions are involved such as the timing, sight of food, the smell, mouth feel and taste. Much of this is tied into social behaviors, and socially condoned behaviors. In the past it was the three martini lunch, the business lunch, a quick stop at Starbuck's, or the "snack" of cheeseburgers, hamburgers and fries and a large soft drink at your favorite fast food restaurant.

For your continuing success with weight loss, and weight management, you will need to exert your own independence and rely on your own motivation to do so. Set realistic goals for yourself, and with the help offered here, you will be better educated and more informed about the control you can exert in your world. Shop to control the kinds of foods that you bring into your home. Become aware of what you eat, and the places that you eat. Sit while eating and do not eat while watching television, the internet or reading. Do you know what is in your refrigerator? Use a refrigerator inventory form to check the foods that you stock in your refrigerator on a regular basis. Remember, each day you are getting more healthy habits and extinguishing the older, unhealthy habits. You are becoming more in control of your situating. Go to the refrigerator with your checklist and look at the items to check everything you have now. Then, reexamine the foods. You will become more aware of the food you eat routinely, and then become more competent at knowing the food that is the healthier alternatives. Once you understand the difference between high calorie and lower calorie, higher fiber foods, you will be better to able minimize your contact with higher calorie, less healthy foods. Minimize your contact with the more processed foods. These are usually higher fat, lower fiber, higher saturated fats, or high in processed carbohydrate content. Most always, they provide more calories than the number of nutrients they contain, making them low nutrient density foods. This is not to say that you cannot buy them, but if you do not buy them routinely, you will not eat them regularly. Setting short term goals, with the end in mind, will make your plan workable.

Food diaries are very popular with nutrition experts because it is proven that when people are watched, questioned and asked to write everything down, food habits are altered. Why? As you become more aware of what you are eating, or you want to avoid writing down foods that you are aware are not helping you to lose weight. Or you may be embarrassed to record it, knowing that your counselor will see what you are eating. However, over time the chore of writing down everything will make you less likely to continue. Today, there are apps that make it much easier to record especially with smart phones exactly what you eat. Just a few of them include MyFitDay, or MyFitPlan, SHealth and any number of others. There is even one that will allow you to take a picture of the foods that you eat, and choose the appropriate number of nutrients these foods provide. The problem then becomes, that you need to remember to record, and to record accurately what you have eaten, whether it's a snack or a meal. This takes effort. What is most important though is that for the first time you will notice. What we know we do will require some sort of decision on our part to continue or to decide to change our habits. Habits once examined can be extinguished. The goal then in weight management is the control of eating habits, examination and improvement of the faulty ones. Less food is needed to control hunger than appetite. Don't eat when you are not hungry. Learn to identify the three types of hunger; situational, emotional and physical. If you decrease your physical exposure to food you will be less likely to be tempted by it. For example, if you are bored, and you get up and go to the kitchen to get a toothpick. You see a partially eaten cake, or your own personal food weakness sitting on the counter, you will have to think about the possibility of having "just a taste". But if the cake was not there in the first place, you might be less apt to think about it. Know what your pitfalls are and at least keep these foods out of sight or even out of your kitchen. Select higher fiber, lower calorie foods and allow yourself a larger portion size. Tomatoes and cucumbers with vinegar or in fact most any fresh vegetables are good snacks. You can have up to three cups of most raw vegetables. Add rice wine vinegar, apple cider vinegar, or lemon juice as an enhancement. Fresh fruits are acceptable, in fact frozen grapes are great, but avoid fruit juice because although they may be unsweetened, the calories can add up too quickly. Eat and drink slowly, and enjoy every taste. Savor each and every morsel. Again, work to plan your eight hours of sleep, particularly in the first few weeks when you are working diligently to develop new habits. You will be less likely to stray from your plans, and yield to temptations when you are not over tired and mentally alert. By getting eight hours of sleep you will be decreasing your gherin level and be less apt to react to stressors during the day. This stress hormone can sabotage your weight loss or management. Finally, think of this time as a learning period for extinguishing the old entrenched habits, and for the development of the new thin eating habits that will become part of the way of life for you. A note about developing new habits; it takes thirteen weeks to develop a new habit.

How much control do you exert over your environment? Analyze again the facts both and pro and con for breakfast in the morning, or the rearrangement of your individual eating pattern. Do try to analyze the places you eat. Have you ever wished you could control your environment?

You can blame the environment and all the other variables that come into play including peer pressure. "Let's have a Big Mac!" You can blame the societal evils, the birthday parties, the cocktail parties, the bachelorette parties, the baby showers, or afternoon tea including all the reasons to celebrate. But when all is said and done, the fact remains that you as a product of your environment must learn to deal with yourself in that environment. We are a society of celebrations set around food. Remember the Christmas that someone made the eggnog too strong? Or the holiday that both Aunt Lee and Aunt Thenis made pumpkin pie and fruitcake? Nothing in your environment is going to change unless you make it change. Change your mindset. If you want to you can! Now, re-examine the list of reasons for wanting to lose weight. Write the reasons down. Do not just think about them. Get out a pen and paper and write. Start with number one and list the reasons you want to lose weight now! Read it and then re-read it over carefully. Have you convinced yourself that you want to lose weight? Good! Now take the responsibility for your own weight state.

Jean Paul Sartre stated, "Man is responsible for what he is and what he becomes in his lifetime." Oh yes, you can blame your fatness on your genes, and in five percent of the cases you will be correct. Remember, though hormonal imbalance is responsible for only five per cent or less of those instances. You can blame your overweight state on your environment and the eating habits that you learned since your birth. There is more truth to that, and familial obesity is responsible for your weight status because eating is a learned response, so here you are probably correct. Studies indicate that families having one obese and one normal weight parent will probably rear an overweight child. This is more probably true when the obese parent is the mother. The family is most affected by the person responsible for buying and preparing the foods served in the household. Were you a member of the "Clean Plate Club"? That is environmental conditioning. But you no longer have to let your environment condition you. Stop immediately and begin to condition your environment. To change the way you interact with food and engineer a skinny environment. Use the checklist, YOU HAVE BEEN EATING WHERE?

One of the most difficult aspects in life is doing something differently for the way it has always been done. A change in your behavior will make for a stressful situation. But stress is not always or only bad. On the other hand, change is only as good as the need to change requires. It is the individual's requirement to change that will dictate the difference in methodology. We all have a routine, when we get up whether it is the early morning, late morning or the late afternoon. We will plug in the coffee, shower, dress, and head for whatever our work is for the day. For only one week change your pattern to include a breakfast food. Notice, I did not say breakfast in the traditional sense. Impossible, you say? Then rethink the possibilities. Embrace a basic premise in control. First change your eating habits, and living pattern. If it didn't work the way you were doing it before, why without change would you believe that it will succeed now? This change is only for one week. If it doesn't work, then go back to the way you were doing things before. Okay? Then give it a try. The first step in this drastic change is to analyze the force behind the change. Why is breakfast or just one breakfast food so important? Your brain uses a simple monosaccharide or sugar, glucose for energy. There is a blood brain barrier and your brain only accepts glucose as its source of energy; not fat, amino acids nor protein. From the time your body stopped eating until the time you awaken you have been in a fasting state. During that time, your body lowered its energy requirements, but when you arise you begin your flurry of activities, and must raise your blood glucose to accommodate the needs and accelerate for the maximum efficiency for your brain. By eating, you are giving your body fuel for energy and you are beginning to promote gastric motility by increasing fiber and liquids in your system. Studies have shown that your initial meal (breaking the fast) increasing your efficiency especially in the midmorning period. So begin everyday with a breakfast food. Include a good source of carbohydrate, protein for satiety value and efficiency, and some fat. Your changed pattern might look something like this; half a cup of plain low fat or nonfat yogurt and fresh seasonal berries, a hard boiled egg, a piece of whole grain high fiber bread, or either a hot or cold cereal such as oatmeal, or shredded wheat. Start off with a glass of eight ounces of cold water, and a small glass of a natural juice, preferably high in Vitamin C. Now, ask yourself the question, why do you skip breakfast? Is it because of time constraints or the time that you would have to get up to implement the breakfast plan? Can you plan to do some of the things that you will need to do in the morning the night before? Maybe lay out your clothes, or prepack your lunch. Dish up your cereal, or your yogurt? Could you set your alarm to allow for a fifteen minute leeway to accomplish the tasks you generally do? Finally, is anyone else up and having breakfast before leaving the house? If you can't seen to get excited about breakfast, even a liquid breakfast Vita mix or similar is better than nothing. Who knows you might even like it.

When do I eat? Engineering a Skinny Environment Checklist

Not all foods are problem foods so begin by making individual lists of foods that appear to be a problem to avoid for you personally.

DAY	1	2	3	4	5	6	7
Shop only with a list							
Shop only after eating. NEVER SHOP WHEN HUNGRY							
Buy hard to prepare rather than easy to eat foods							
Keep all food stored out of sight							
No salt or high calorie condiments On the table							
No serving dishes on the table							
Clean plates and put remains in The garbage. NO NIBBLES							
Cover leftovers in serving dishes And refrigerate for another meal							
Serve foods in measured portions							
Avoid the purchase of problem foods							
If you do buy problem foods then Prepare them in small batches							
Instead of storing problem foods in the Refrigerator, go out for a treat; ice cream Cone versus a quart of ice cream in the freezer							
Leave the table when you are finished							

Food out of sight means temptation out of reach.

When you need more support go to www.notimefordiets.com

Chapter 11

CANDLELIGHT FOR TWO...
Holiday and Restaurant Dining

The lights are low...its, finally just the two of you, after a hectic day, a harried week, a frustrating month. There's no reason for restraint. This opportunity may not happen again, right?

"Wrong!" This moment is what you make it and not what food makes it. A great meal does not make or break an evening. A wonderful evening is had, in spite of a disgusting meal and conversely, a wonderful meal, makes a disgusting evening slightly more bearable.

"Yes. Restaurant dining does present a challenge." But it can spell success while you maintain some semblance of sanity. Here's how. Set your own limits before you go out and follow your plan. Make it a point to drink one or two glasses of water before the meal. This will give your sensor receptors a chance to begin working towards that twenty minutes while you are having your appetizers, or cocktail. It's imperative that you work out the type of meal that you can eat without confusion. If you know you are going to exceed your limit know why. Order what? Order a la carte. Diet items are noted on menus but not always. This works especially well with breakfast in Mexican menu items.

Pre-plan! Fast food restaurants are the most expensive calorie wise and unfortunately comprise over 45% of all eating places in the United States. As far back as 1981, McDonalds spent $322 million in advertising. A lot you say? Then consider that their sales exceeded $7 billion dollars. Over the years we have consumed 452% more frozen potatoes, 119% more hard cheeses, and 222% more soft drinks. What do restaurants and fast food drives through restaurants have that we don't need? Calories; A Big Mac French fried and a shake will top 1170 Calories. Wendy's double cheeseburger fries and a shake will provide 1516 Calories. More than that; you will need half of the Calories recommended by the RDI to get only one third of the nutrients you need. In these restaurants 40-50% of the calories come from fat. Don't forget about sodium. The recommended intake is less than 2000 milligrams daily. Please be on the alert, as the sodium in foods increases, the company may list sodium in grams. There are 1000 milligrams in one gram. Call the restaurant before you make your reservations to find out what is available on the menu. Choose a restaurant that offers a good variety of foods. This makes the selection easier. Choosing from a menu that includes a salad bar is a lot easier than from one that specializes in fried foods. A word or two must be said about salads and the salad bars that are so popular in restaurants today. They are truly extensive, and you could actually have your entire meal from the salad selections. Avoid Cole slaw or similar side dishes that have the dressing mixed in. They add extra fat calories that you don't want to deal with. Use a side dish for the dressing. Avoid placing the dressing directly on your salad. If you order a salad to be served at the table, ask for the dressing to be served on the side. That way, you, not the server has control of the amount of fat that you need to have on a salad. Ask for extra vinegar or lemon juice. You can dilute the calories of the dressing almost by half and still retain the original flavor. Ask for a wedge of lemon, and squeeze it over the salad for added flavor without the unwanted fat calories. Once you have the dressing in a side dish, beware of the way you serve yourself. Remember that one teaspoon is considered a fat exchange, and that is equivalent of 50 calories or more, usually not less. Try this first. Dip your fork in the side dish and then into the salad. The amount that you have on your fork will be small but enough to flavor the entire bite of salad. After you have finished using this method, note the amount of salad dressing that is still remaining in the side dish. Just for fun, measure how many teaspoons of fat at fifty calories a teaspoon you saved. "Applause, please!"

Remember that your budgeted calories do add up. Foods served with extra large portions have meats untrimmed, and with added sauces and gravies. Vegetables are served with butter and sauces. Ask for your doggies' bag first. It is so much less tempting to place the extra out of sight and out of mind before you have even tasted the fare. You can even find something that will work into your meal pattern in a Mexican or Chinese restaurant if the selection is extensive enough. Many restaurants, trains, and planes will make modified items available, especially when given some advance notice. In medium priced restaurants, foods can be ordered if requested. Portion sizes are large, and meats and poultry usually have fat untrimmed. Think small and order a single hamburger instead of a double cheeseburger. Order a cup of soup rather than a bowl. Consider ordering half orders of sandwiches, or share your portion with a friend. Sauces or gravies may come on the entree, so be sure to ask for the accompaniments, sauces, gravy, butter, sour cream, and salad dressings on the side. In more expensive restaurants, food prepared as ordered is most always available. Fresh vegetables can be cooked to order, and steamed without butter, or salt. Oriental restaurants are almost always higher in sodium especially if they use MSG. Inexpensive restaurants and fast food restaurants are usually the most expensive calorie-wise. Stick to roasts and baked potatoes to avoid excessive amounts of sodium and fat. Mixers for the cocktails while waiting for your table should be water, rocks, diet soda, or club soda. Since wines are the lowest in calories, choose a white or red wine. Avoid milk shakes, chocolate milk, cocoa, or soft drinks, unless its water. Dietetic sodas have their own problems. The artificial sweetener will often trick your metabolism

Carry your own Stevia. Then, if there is a paucity of sugar substitutes you have yours. Remember, you have a budget to follow, and the calories will add up. Why waste your calories on something as unimportant as sugar. In one single teaspoon, there are twenty "empty" calories. Calories that are nearly devoid of nutrients. If you use two or three teaspoons of sugar in your coffee, or tea, that adds up to forty or sixty calories. Maybe I'm being measly, but it's true. Persnickety, perhaps! But a calorie saved is a calorie burned!

Where do you eat? Select a restaurant that serves simple foods that are cooked to order. When you dine out daily, it's wise to select a specific restaurant. Your food is more likely to receive special attention if you're a regular customer.

Foods are usually served in extra sized portions. (8-16 ounces) with meats untrimmed, and salads served with the dressing applied, in most instances. Learn to judge portion sizes by practicing at home. Knowing what a four ounce portion of meat or chicken or one cup of rice looks like, or one teaspoon of dressing makes "guesstimating" portions at restaurants easier. Ask questions about the portion sizes and how the food is prepared. Just how big is a medium pizza? How many ounces of meat in my steak? Does the taco come with guacamole? Vegetables are usually seasoned with butter, or a sauce with some fat added or a cheese sauce applied.

How can you guard against this onslaught of blessings from the manufacturer our "God of Plenty"? It's imperative that you work out the type of meal that you can eat without confusion. Remember the phrase is "without confusion". If you know that you're going to exceed your limit, know why. It's okay to put yourself in debt if you know what you're going to do to compensate for it and get yourself back on track again with more exercise. Ask for a "doggie bag" even before you begin. Not to posh you say? Extremely posh, I say. If you must, explain that you are under the supervision of a Nutritionist who cautions you not to eat more than six ounces of protein daily due to renal overload. Now, when the entree is served, USE that doggie bag before you begin. Why? Because, that, my dear, is the fun of a gourmet restaurant. You may want to continue to eat, far beyond the point that your sensory receptors have given you the message that the amount is sufficient and you are satisfied. It's less tempting to place the extra out of sight, before you taste the fare. There have been many times that I have used the doggie bag and never carried it from the table. That worked out well too. You will not overeat, yet you can totally enjoy the food that is placed before you and half of today's meal can be tomorrow's lunch. You'll have planned for your next day's meal, saving time, money, and calories.

Order what? Order a la carte. Diet items noted on menus are not always low in calories. This works especially well at breakfast meals, or at Mexican restaurants. The extras come in a complete meal costs you extra money and calories. For appetizers, order tea, vegetable juices (note that they may be higher in sodium, unsweetened juices (count them as a choice from the allowed fruits), broth, consommé or bouillon (high sodium). Fresh vegetables; celery, radishes, broccoli are good dippers with a plain, low fat yogurt.

Avoid ordering cream soups, soups with rice or barley unless you count the pasta as part of your starch allowance. Finally, only order a fish or meat appetizer if you are planning to reduce the size of the entree.

Entrees of stewed, roasted, simmered, barbequed, poached or broiled fish make the safest choice. Chicken, or beef with skin removed or fat trimmed are next best. If you order fried, sautéed, breaded or casserole, you have to think of the added choices that you are using. Don't order bacon wrapped meats, and gravies should always be ordered on the side because to the added fat. Two ounces of gravy contains two fat choices plus one bread choice, or 18 grams of fat. That adds up to one hundred and sixty-two calories from fat. Avoid fried or scrambled eggs. If you order grilled items place them on a napkin to remove much of the fat. Ordering potatoes? Keep it plain, or order two vegetables instead. Oder baked, boiled, or steamed. Avoid home fries, French fries, browned, creamed, scalloped or mashed. Beware of sweetened or frosted breads. After making your selection, ask the waiter or your companion to place the rolls out of reach to avoid further temptation. Use bacon, cream and butter in small amounts. Request vinegar, and lemon for your salad choices and fresh fruit salads count as part of the choices for fruit for the day. If you order Cole slaw you need to think about the fat because of the mayonnaise used. Check vegetables as they may have butter added without your knowledge. Ask the waiter and if he seems uninformed, proceed with the knowledge that they have probably had butter added.

Ah, yes. Dessert!! Delay or eat it later, at home. If you do order have fresh fruit. Beware of pies, custard, or cakes. Drink your coffee or tea plain or use your Stevia as a sugar substitute. Then relax and enjoy the company of your meal companions. Make them the focus of the mealtime, not the food.

The Fourth of July, or any holiday is a time of celebration. Let go! Have the time of your life. It is also a time when our daily routines are upset. Our time schedule and time with family members has a slightly less well defined time schedule. Our eating styles change and the "what the heck" and "just this once" attitudes prevail. We tend to overindulge, feel guilty, and plan to starve ourselves after the holidays are over.

What about a new strategy this year? Holidays spell buffets, some of everything, and party, party, party! Instead of eating everything, eat a little of your favorites. There are many levels between self deprivation, and overindulgence. The main objective is to PLAN, PLAN, and PLAN! What usually happens during the holidays? Where are your weaknesses? Avoid and work around and away from your weaknesses avoid getting caught in the old impulse habit. While making plans for gifts, and guests, make some plans for yourself as well. By thinking ahead you will have a greater tendency to follow that plan instead of being led by the impulse, or old habits. Set a realistic goal for yourself. Instead of planning to lose weight during the holidays this is a great time to maintain the status quo. Plan to maintain your weight. That is the most practical approach. And when you sit down and think about it, and review the stress test, almost any holiday situation will put you in a situation that is not appropriate for weight loss. Holidays spell buffet style dining in many instances. Instead of eating some of everything, plan to take a few of your favorites, in moderate amounts. Many people pile their plates high out of habit. Your eyes are bigger than your stomach, and then these same people try to stretch their stomach to match. Eat slowly, enjoy what you are eating. Then, remember to have that eight ounces of cold water and take the twenty minutes for your sensor receptors. Enjoy the company and social situation of the meal. Focus on the people and the pleasure of the company and less on the food as the source of pleasure. Special people are what make this a special celebration. Plan for established meal times, to avoid the "snacking all day" syndrome. You might consider preparing meals in advance if you know that you are going to be busy. Allow yourself one planned treat, and enjoy that. Establish a "splurge" allowance. Then its legal and you won't need to binge. Plan activities to keep busy and away from the kitchen or center of the foods. Walks are great to help work off extra calories and the children will think that it's a treat. You may find that you actually enjoy getting some fresh air. When purchasing food for guests, buy in small quantities. This will allow for the extra piece of pie that Uncle Gus didn't finish. Have enough low calorie foods on hand for yourself and others to munch on. You'd be surprised how many people are watching the amounts that they eat, and will appreciate your concern. How about a low calorie dip and fresh vegetables? It doesn't have to taste low calorie. Stay away from holiday treats, and for example, one instead of two cookies, and a small piece of pumpkin pie. Now that's planning. Keep tempting foods out of sight. If leftover dressing is your nemesis, store in a covered container, and keep it out of sight. The less visual cues you have, the less likely that you will be to respond.

Think small! Bake tarts, not pies, half a batch of cookies. If you love to bake, donate your baked goods to a church or bake sale. Keep a large glass of cold water in an attractive holiday mug within reach when you feel the urge to munch. Sometimes, all you need is a drink to hold and socialize with. Use these suggestions as a basis and then be creative. Now, deck the halls with boughs of holly, stand under a sprig of mistletoe and get ready to enjoy the holidays!

The following exercises are to help to uncover the double entendres of food. These are ways that food can and has become tied into thoughts of times without even your realizing that you are beginning to develop an appetite for our favorite foods through celebrations. First, think of a particular food that you cannot eat because it is absolutely distasteful. Now think back to the first and last times that you ate or encountered the food. What situations were associated with the particular food?

What foods or food do you particularly associate with Thanksgiving? Most would say that's obvious, a big tom turkey, but others might have answers that are entirely different, because of family traditions that have developed through the years. What would happen if those foods were absent on Thanksgiving? When purchasing food for guests buy in small quantities. This will allow for the extra piece of pies that Uncle Gus didn't finish. Have enough low calorie foods to munch on. You may be surprised at how many others are watching what they eat and will be thankful for the consideration. How about low calorie dip and fresh vegetables? It doesn't have to taste low calorie. Now think of the foods most closely associated with Christmas. Do you associate any foods with a particular holiday activity? For example do you think of hot chocolate and caroling? Be sure that its sugar free! Remember having Eggnog around a fireside, or at New Years holidays? Think small, instead of a huge mug, how about a demitasse. Bake tarts not pies, and half batch of cookies, or donate the extras to the bake sale or church. Keep a large glass of low calorie beverage in an attractive holiday mug within reach when you feel the urge to sip or munch. Use these suggestions as a basis and then be creative. Now deck the halls with boughs of holly, and stand under a sprig of mistletoe to get ready to rock!

Think of a particular vacation spot, and a food associated with it; for example, picture a Down East paradise and a lobster or steamed clam dinner. Remember to change the picture to a more healthful food if necessary. For example, you might want to change a baked stuffed lobster to a boiled live one, or a fried clam dinner to a steamed clam feast! Break state. Take a five minute break or longer. Do something that will totally change your attitude. If you take time to feel good about yourself, you will begin to feel good in general. Do not feel guilty for taking time for yourself. If you don't love yourself, the no one else will relate to you. Keep an active mind. Do not sit and think about how difficult it is not to think about food. Choose something else to think about. Find a better substitute and focus on that. Try different hobbies, and read for enjoyment. Inside of you is a person that you want to be. Be that person. Let that inner person surface. Self criticism is forbidden here. We are not looking for perfection, just improvement. Reject the idea of the status quo! Keep the good thoughts. Simply get rid of the calories